Praise for REBUILT

"A deeply enjoyable book. Chorost ponders what is 'real' to us in our natural state and what our 'natural' state really is, and how what is real to us will change over time, and thus change us."

—RODNEY BROOKS, director of the MIT Computer Science and Artificial Intelligence Lab

"A compelling and sensitive account of life as a 'cyborg.'"

—*Reader's Digest*, Editor's Choice

"Chorost's graceful, poetic turns of phrase and dry, self-deprecating humor take what could have been a dry technological story and breathe life into it . . . this is a book that will make you think and, ultimately, make you smile." —*Library Journal*, starred review

"Engagingly geeky, unafraid to delve into his intimate medical details, dating catastrophes, and TV fixations, Michael Chorost brings a new technological twist to the modern memoir." —*Seattle Weekly*

"The most hopeful thing I've read in quite a while."

—*San Francisco Bay Guardian*

"Chorost makes the complexities of the [cochlear implant] system clear . . . but it is the technology's human depth that he mines to best effect."

—*Buffalo News*

"Remarkable and warmly funny." —*East Bay Express*

"A heartfelt exploration of technologically mediated perception and the impact of a cochlear implant on one man's experience and sense of self. Chorost's journey is that of humanity itself."

—ANDY CLARK, author of *Natural-Born Cyborgs*

"A quite amazing new writer whose prose spirits the reader across the sound barrier from deafness to a new world."

—SOL STEIN, author of *Stein on Writing*

"An artfully frank account, Chorost's story will vitally engage people interested in the increasingly prevalent surgical procedure." —*Booklist*

"[Chorost] recounts with candor and humor his struggles with relationships, both casual and intimate . . . in this beautifully written debut."

—*Publishers Weekly*

Rebuilt

MY JOURNEY BACK TO THE HEARING WORLD

Michael Chorost

A MARINER BOOK
Houghton Mifflin Company
BOSTON • NEW YORK

First Mariner Books edition 2006

Visit our Web site: www.houghtonmifflinbooks.com.

The Library of Congress has cataloged the hardcover edition as follows:

Chorost, Michael.
Rebuilt : how becoming part computer made me more human / Michael Chorost.
p. cm.
Includes bibliographical references and index.
ISBN 0-618-37829-4
Cochlear implants—Patients—United States—Biography.
I. Title.
RF305.C465 2005 617.8'8220592'092—dc22
[B] 2005040335

ISBN-13: 978-0-618-71760-6 (pbk.)
ISBN-10: 0-618-71760-9 (pbk.)

Printed in the United States of America

Book design by Robert Overholtzer

QUM 10 9 8 7 6 5 4 3 2 1

Illustration credits: Figures 2, 3, and 9: Photos courtesy Advanced Bionics. Figure 4: Photo copyright © Mikhail Lemkhin. Figures 6 and 7: Images courtesy Elsevier and James O. Pickles. Reprinted from *An Introduction to the Physiology of Hearing*, 2nd ed., James O. Pickles, pages 33 and 300. Copyright © 1988, with permission from Elsevier. Figure 8 is based on a graph provided by Robert Shannon, House Ear Institute, Los Angeles, California.

TO THE SCIENTISTS, ENGINEERS, SURGEONS,
AUDIOLOGISTS, and CLINICAL-TRIAL PATIENTS
who contributed to developing the cochlear
implant over forty years of research and labor,
this book is dedicated in humility
and admiration.

AND TO MOM AND DAD,
my first and best teachers.

The poet will naturally write about that which most deeply engrosses him — and nothing more deeply engrosses a man than his burdens, including those of a physical nature, such as disease. We win by capitalizing on our debts, by turning our liabilities into assets, by using our burdens as a basis of insight.

—Kenneth Burke, *The Philosophy of Literary Form*

"Gentlemen, we can rebuild him."

—Voice-over opening of *The Six Million Dollar Man*

Contents

1. Broken

I'M IMPATIENT. It hasn't been a good morning. I'm on a business trip and have just arrived in Reno, where I'm supposed to interview people at Tahoe for a study. But the car rental at the airport won't take my debit card. I spend half an hour canvassing the other outlets, no luck. Finally a man at one counter kindly names a competitor and points me to a courtesy phone.

"Dial 133. They usually have cars and their rates are okay."

I pick up the phone. I can hear it fine with my hearing aids, even amid the ruckus of the baggage claim. Yes, they have cars available. The voice directs me to the shuttle bus outside the airport.

It's the last telephone call I will ever make with my natural ears.

Paperwork signed, I wait for my car. I fidget. I might as well have driven here instead of flying. And then —

That's odd. The traffic sounds fuzzy all of a sudden. Instead of their usual decisive *vrump,* the cars have started making a whispery sound as they go by, as if plowing through shredded paper. And they sound a hundred yards away, even though I'm right by the road.

It sounds like my left hearing aid's battery is going. Even though I'm wearing two hearing aids, only the left ear really counts. The right ear is so poor that it can hear only vague rumbles. My left ear is my conversation ear, my telephone ear, my radio ear.

I switch batteries in a practiced little *pas de deux* of the hands: left battery into the right aid, right battery into the left. That doesn't make any difference. I guess they're *both* going. I pull out a battery pack from my suitcase, do a second changeout, and wait for the familiar rush of clean, loud sound. But it doesn't happen.

I can't have two broken hearing aids at once. It's as absurd as two tires blowing out at the same time. As I get in the car I'm breathing shallowly, and it's not because of the altitude. I roll the car window down, fiddle with my left hearing aid's volume control, and wait for my ears to miraculously clear. All the way up to Tahoe, I'm monitoring on all frequencies, and — *this doesn't sound right.*

Gotta be the batteries. It's just a pack of bad batteries. At the hotel I check in, then go to the Long's drugstore and buy three sets of 675s. It costs me fifteen dollars and thirty-seven cents. Right there at the checkout counter, I rip the batteries out of their plastic case and put them in.

That doesn't help either.

In the car I spread both hearing aids out on the passenger seat and methodically try every possible combination of tubes, batteries, and earmolds. Nothing works: the day is like a coin that always comes up tails.

"It's got to be earwax," I say to myself out loud, looking out the windshield at the big red-and-white logo of the store.

I've got to get someone to check my left ear for earwax. Maybe the clerk at the hotel? She had proved to be a lissome woman with blond hair layered over black, whose full lips pouted as her hands explored a keyboard I couldn't see. Maybe she would also take me into her arms and tell me that everything would be all right. Now *that* would be customer service.

I've never had earwax trouble in my life. But I've also never had two hearing aids fail on me at once, either.

Emergency room. Now.

The ER is quiet, so while waiting for the doctor I conduct an impromptu interview with the nurse. The study is on the region's social problems, and I might as well start collecting data. The nurse is a fount of information. But as she talks, a chilly realization takes hold of me.

"Nancy," I say. "Are you talking about as loudly as you were when I first came in?"

"Yes, I think so."

"But I'm not hearing you as well as when I came in. Before, I could mostly hear your voice. Now I'm only getting little bits of it."

I'm having to lip-read her more and more. With perceptible speed, the world is becoming softer and softer. Every half-hour, I am hearing less than the half-hour before. It's like being an astronaut in the movie *Apollo 13* watching the oxygen tank's gauge inexorably sliding down to zero.

Reflexively, I think to myself: *It's the battery.*

Oh no it isn't. I have not only just lost part of my hearing, I am losing all of it. Minute by minute. I am going completely deaf, right here, right now, while sitting on this table talking to this nurse and scribbling notes.

The nurse goes off to see if she can find the physician just a little bit sooner. In a few minutes he appears, listens grave-faced to my story, then looks carefully in my ears.

"Your ears both look the same," he tells me after I put my hearing aids back in. "There's no fluid behind the eardrums. No redness or swelling."

I can barely hear him, even though I've twisted the volume wheels on both my aids up to max. I usually set the volume at three. Now it's at five, the top number on the dial. I need it to be at *six.* Six is my world of a few hours ago, the place where footsteps and birds and telephones live. If I could just get it to *six.*

"I'm also feeling a little dizzy," I say cautiously, knowing the implications but trying not to think about them. The inner ears also control the sense of balance. I feel lightheaded, off-kilter, ethereal, as if I had just downed a shot of vodka. When I'd gotten off the exam bench to greet the doctor I had first looked down at the floor to check how far away it was. On the fly, I'm reorganizing the way

I deal with my visual field. I'm finding that if I turn to look at something too fast, my head swims. To stop that from happening, I've started squinting and holding my eyes steady as I turn my head.

The doctor goes off to call a specialist. I peer around the curtain to watch him at the nurses' station down the hall. The phone's spiral cord skitters over the counter as he paces back and forth.

He comes back, speaking slowly and carefully so I can read his lips. "It could be a virus in the inner ear. I want to prescribe you steroids and antivirals. They treat swelling caused by viruses like herpes —"

I'm unraveling his words one at a time, and this creates a kind of myopia of the soul. The words are roaming around in my brain and not slotting in anywhere.

"*Herpes?* I don't have herpes."

"It's not that. It's an *antiviral*."

Steroids. Antivirals. Vertigo. It is sinking into me that this is not earwax, this is not an equipment problem, this is not a minor health scare. I am in deep trouble. My mission is aborted. My life has changed forever. *Six* is lost, unreachable, in a place beyond where the volume wheel stops. Whip right around Tahoe, take the fastest trajectory back home.

The day is July 7, 2001. I'm thirty-six years old. I've just finished my Ph.D. After a decade of grad school I'm learning what it's like to have a real job and the beginning of a career. I'm starting to meet people. I'm beginning to have a life.

I have always been hard of hearing. That's not the same thing as being deaf. To be hard of hearing is to have partial hearing, which my hearing aids remedied by amplifying sound. They hurt, itched, and whistled, yet they enabled me to take my place in a hearing world. I went to school with people who heard normally. I could use the telephone and understand the radio. No one ever taught me sign language. I often stumbled; I had to ask for repeats; I constantly missed jokes and struggled at parties; but I got by, a reasonably successful child of a lesser god.

I've always been hard of hearing. I can't go *deaf.**

Not *now.*

Eight hours later I return to the car rental office only to find it closed and deserted. A sign directs me to deposit the key and call for a courtesy cab. A yellow arrow points helpfully to the location of the phone. I go and stare at it, feeling like Snoopy in a world filled with signs saying NO DOGS ALLOWED. The lot is vacant, not a human being in sight. What do I do?

Perhaps I have *just* enough hearing left to hear a yes. I pick up the phone and dial.

"Mmmm mmm mmbpm bbmm verumf hmm bmm, berum hmmm hmm-hmmm grmmm."

"Hi, I'm at the Enterprise Rent-a-car lot and I need a ride to the airport. The sign says to call. Can you send a cab?"

"Erumm vrmm nerpmm mmm mmbpm ermm bmmm arimm, mmmbpmm bmm hmm ermmm —"

"I'm sorry, I'm deaf and I can't hear you. Could you just say *yes* or *no*? Just say whether you can send a cab. Just one word, please. I'm at the Enterprise Rent-a-car near the Reno airport, on" — I look around desperately, my ears ringing like chimes as my head swivels — "Mill Road."

"*Ssssss* burumm bmm pmmb erumm bmm pmm arumm emm er berumm bmm pmm bmm erumm burumm."

Human beings are not binary creatures. You can ask as clearly as possible for a single syllable, *yes* or *no*, 1 or 0, but the instinctual apparatus of social communication is not easily turned off. Even audiologists will blather on at me while they are holding my hearing aids in their own hands, and I have to smile tolerantly and hold up my hand to stop them. To people who hear normally, complete

* The word *deaf* is fraught with definitional and political complexities. Just as many "blind" people still have some vision, many "deaf" people still have some hearing. Audiologists therefore prefer to use the terms *hard of hearing* and *hearing-impaired.* Conversely, many members of the signing deaf community use the capitalized word *Deaf* to distinguish themselves from non-signers, whom they consider merely "deaf." I find terms like *hard of hearing* awkward to use repeatedly, so from this point on I will usually use the term *deaf* to describe myself.

deafness seems to be inconceivable. Complete blindness can be simulated easily by closing one's eyes, but even the best earplugs cannot fully shut out the world. The ears are always on, always connected. To talk is to be heard.

But I have gotten just enough of the sibilant, the *ssss* in *yes,* to get the message. "Okay, I hear you saying *yes,* thank you, I'll wait for the cab."

I hang up, praying that all the phonic baggage trailing that one syllable was not *yes, but it will take an hour,* or *yes, but you have to call this other number,* or *yes, we will send a cab right away, sir, if you would just say again where you are.*

I stand there and wait, clutching the tow handle of my suitcase as the sun pivots and falls, as appalled by the enormity of the parking lot as a castaway who has just watched his last message in a bottle drift out of sight.

In the maze of doctors' visits that take place in the next few weeks, a phrase that comes up over and over again is *cochlear implant.* When people go deaf, it is usually because something is wrong with a snail-shaped organ called the *cochlea,* which lives behind the eardrum, about an inch and a half inside the skull. (The word *cochlea* comes from the Latin word for "snail.") The entire function of the rest of the ear — the ear canal, the eardrum, the three little bones of the middle ear — is just to get sound to the cochlea. The ear canal funnels sound toward the eardrum, which vibrates. Three little bones transmit the eardrum's vibration to the base of the cochlea (that is, the big end of its spiral). Ripples travel through the fluid inside the cochlea from its base to the apex. As they go, they perturb 15,000 cell-sized hairs lining its inside. Seen at magnification, those hairs look like a field of grass, and in fact they behave like one, literally rustling in response to sound waves just as blades of grass undulate to the wind's touch. Each hair is connected to a nerve ending, which sends signals to the brain when the hair is moved by sound.

If *all* of the hairs are physically damaged — and that appears to be what has just happened to me — the nerves can no longer be stimulated, and profound deafness sets in. But the nerves themselves are usually still intact, and can be triggered with implanted electrodes under computer control. That is what a cochlear implant does.*

Becky Highlander, my new audiologist, explains to me how it works. She's a slender blond woman with a direct gaze and a deadpan sense of humor. Lip-reading her is not so hard right now, because I've been all over the Web researching the device and already have the big picture. Holding up one of the implants, she tells me that the process would start with sound going into the microphone at the headpiece. The headpiece would stick to my head, held there by a magnet inside the implant. The microphone would convert sound into electrical current and send it down a wire running under my shirt to a waist-worn computer (or *processor*) on my belt. The processor would analyze the sound, ultimately yielding a stream of bits (1s and 0s). It would send those bits back up the wire to the headpiece, which would then transmit them by radio through my skin to the computer chips in the implant.

Those chips would send signals down a wire going to my cochlea through a tunnel drilled through an inch and a half of bone. A string of sixteen electrodes coiled up inside my cochlea would strobe on and off in rapid sequence to trigger my auditory nerves. If all went well, my brain would learn to interpret the stimulation as sound.

Getting the implant would make me, in the most literal sense, a *cyborg*. The word is shorthand for *cyb*ernetic *org*anism, a term coined by Manfred Clynes and Nathan Kline in 1960 and defined by WordNet as "a human being whose body has been taken over in whole or in part by electromechanical devices." The word *cybernetic* comes from the Greek *kubernetes,* meaning "pilot" or "steersman." A thermostat is a simple cybernetic device, turning on the heat

* See the Appendix for a diagram of the ear and the components of a cochlear implant.

when temperatures get low and turning it off when they get high. It monitors the world and exerts control on it. It makes decisions.

The *cybernetic organism:* me and my steersman, fused together.

But it's not the prospect of surgery that upsets me. What upsets me, considerably, is what's inside the implant. Becky hands me one with its ceramic casing removed. I cradle it in my palm, surprised by its solidness and heft. It's a circuit board, plain and simple. With computer chips. There are clearly hundreds of thousands of transistors in the thing.

It really *is* a computer. It's cold, angular, and digital, yet it's going to be embedded in my flesh, which is warm, squishy, and wet — how is that even *possible?* How can a joining like that not obscurely but permanently *hurt,* the body and brain outraged by the alien language of 0 and 1?

"Sleep on it," Becky says, kindly.

I do, and I dream that I am walking over a dimly lit landscape of tall grass, my body floating several inches into the air with each step as if I am on the moon. I trip and fall, and my head strikes the ground. A computer chip hiding in the scrub senses its opportunity and lances into my head like a bullet. I get up, hand clutching my skull where it entered, and I am dazed and uncertain: what have I just become?

A cyborg. Not the Hollywood kind, but a real one nonetheless. Steve Austin, the test pilot in *The Six Million Dollar Man* who was rebuilt with two bionic legs, a bionic arm, and a bionic eye, is a cyborg from the outside in, with a powerful mechanical body. But this technology would make me a cyborg from the inside out, because the computer would decide what I heard and how I heard it. It would be physically small, but its *effect* on me would be huge. It would be the sole mediator between the auditory world and myself. Since I would hear nothing but what its software allowed, the computer's control over my hearing would be complete.

In a sense, the process would be a reconstruction of my entire body. To be sure, I would still be nearsighted, still brown-haired, still delighted by chocolate and allergic to sesame seeds. But the sense of hearing immerses you in the world as no other. John Hull, a blind man, writes that while the eyes put you at the periphery of the universe — you are always at its edge, looking in — the ears put you at its center, since you hear what is all around you. Hearing constitutes your sense of being *of* the world, in the thick of it. To see is to observe, but to hear is to be enveloped. People who go completely deaf often report feeling dead, invisible, insubstantial. They feel that it is *they* who have become unreal, not the world.

If deafness is a kind of death, hearing again is a kind of rebirth. But I would be reborn into a different body. Becky carefully explains to me that the implant can't restore the living organ in all its subtlety and complexity. The world mediated by the computer in my skull would sound synthetic, the product of approximations, interpolations, and compromises. My body would have bewildering new properties and new rules, and it would take me weeks, months, even years, to understand them fully.

And those properties would keep changing. This new ear would have thousands of lines of code telling it what to do with incoming sound and how to trigger my nerve endings. That code could be changed in two ways. Its settings could be tweaked in a process called *mapping,* which would be a bit like changing Word's font sizes and colors for better readability. Or scientists could change the underlying algorithms themselves as they learned more about how normal ears encode sound for the brain. That would require wiping out the processor's software and replacing it with an entirely new version. It would be the equivalent of changing a computer's operating system from DOS to Windows, or Windows to Linux. My perception of the world would always be provisional: the *latest* but never the *final* version.

Who has not wondered what it would be like to live in someone else's body? If I got the implant, I would find out. An artificial sense organ makes your body *literally* someone else's, perceiving the world by a programmer's logic and rules instead of the ones biology and evolution gave you. "You will be assimilated," the gaunt, riven "Borg" villains of *Star Trek* told their victims. While the implant would not of course control my mind, in a very real sense I *would* be assimilated. A cochlear implant has a corporate mind, created by squadrons of scientists, audiologists, programmers, and clinical-trial patients. I would be *in-corporated,* bound for life to a particular company's changing beliefs in the nature of reality. Resistance would be futile. Unless, of course, I wanted to be deaf.

In 1802, Ludwig van Beethoven wrote to his brothers about the perplexities of deafness.

> My misfortune is doubly painful to me because I am bound to be misunderstood; for me there can be no relaxation with my fellow men, no refined conversations, no mutual exchange of ideas. I must live almost alone, like one who has been banished. I can mix with society only as much as true necessity demands. If I approach near to people a hot terror seizes upon me, and I fear being exposed to the danger that my condition might be noticed.

"No refined conversations," indeed. I had loved to listen to my massage therapist's gentle voice as her hands worked my shoulders and arms. Now that I am completely deaf I just have to lie there, wandering in the dullness of my ingrown mind, while her hands probe my skin. When I am face up things are easier, though being prone, without my glasses, in low light, is not the best conversational situation. The results are atrocious:

"So what have you done this week, Wendy?"

"Mnnn gnorm erumm brmm parumm gerumm."

I crane my head up to look at her. I do my best to repeat what I think I have heard back to her, to save her the trouble of saying it again. "Sandwich?" I realize as I say it that it is a ridiculous guess.

"Mnnn gnorm erumm brmmm party gerumm."

"Party. You had a party?"

"Yes. For Aiyana."

I know that Aiyana is one of the associates of the clinic. At least now I'm contextualized. I can decode better.

"A big party?"

"Serrum gvrmmm."

"Small party?"

"Sixteen. It was just enough."

"Sixteen people. That's a lot for a small space like this." Absurdly, I am assuming she had the party in the office.

"No, at home."

"Ah, at home." I let my head drop back on the table. "I'm sorry I missed it."

It is like returning to the ancient days of 300-baud modems, when one could see text appearing on the screen letter by letter. I communicate phoneme by phoneme, with tin cans and string.

And there are many other little humiliations. I forget to take my change at the supermarket and the bagger runs after me in the parking lot, calling, but I don't turn around until he taps my shoulder. In doctors' offices, I have to apologetically ask receptionists to come and get me when I am called. I don't dare to start conversations with people I don't know.

I'm still able to get things done at work, since most of my job consists of writing anyway. But when I try to attend a meeting with two other people, I can't swivel my head back and forth fast enough to follow what either of them is saying. At first they gamely try to include me, but it's hopelessly tedious and soon they return to doing what they know how to do, which is talk like normal people. They aren't being unkind; they just don't know what more they can do, and neither do I. For about ten minutes I watch them, feeling like HAL, the hyperintelligent computer in Kubrick's *2001,* spying on two astronauts by lip-reading their conversation through a space pod's window. Maybe HAL could do such a thing, but I can't. I see their lips move, I know megabytes of information are flowing back and forth, but it's as invisible to me as radio waves. Finally I quietly excuse myself and they nod me out.

I relinquish my lead responsibilities in the Tahoe contract, turn it over to my supervisor, move to a secondary job devising the survey instruments and doing the background research. It would have been so much fun to barnstorm Tahoe, interviewing anyone who would stand still long enough. That's all impossible now.

Using the telephone is out of the question. And this is the worst limitation of all, because it contracts my social universe into my line of sight. The phone used to be a gateway onto an unseen world of distant family and friends. I can still pick up the handset and put it to my ear, but nothing happens when I do. I can't even hear the dial tone.

But, grotesquely, I am not living in the silent world that I might have expected. That would at least have been familiar, for I had always been able to take my hearing aids out and experience near-total silence. Now, I am living in an endless cacophony. Now I hear a thunderous river, now a jet engine, now a restaurant with a thousand patrons all talking at once. The sound is unending and overwhelming. Silence is the one thing I never have.

No one can really explain to me what is causing the "noise." One theory is that in the total absence of sound, the auditory cortex hallucinates in an attempt to make up for the deficit. Amputees have phantom limb; perhaps I have phantom ear. Another theory is that it is the auditory equivalent of chronic pain, where my damaged cochlea is wildly firing nerve impulses unrelated to sensory stimuli. For hours on end I hear *bing-bing-bing* sounds like the bells at railroad crossings. I can hardly help but interpret it as my ear crying *alarm! alarm! alarm! alarm!*

But there are consolations. In the evenings the rumbles and bells soften. They become grand, sonorous, and deep. I hear a vast organ playing a slowly evolving dirge without a time or a beat. It has the solemn grandeur of an aurora. Occasionally it rises to sustained pitches, like the voiceless wail of Gyorgi Ligeti's *Atmospheres* when the planets come into alignment in *2001*. It fits the occasion, for in 2001 my ears are dying. But they are playing superbly at their own funeral.

It's not only my body and world I can't recognize. I can't even recognize *myself*. Two days after I return from Tahoe, a neurotologist writes me a prescription for an even larger dose of steroids to reduce inflammation in my ears and tells me solemnly, "Don't make any major life decisions while you're taking this stuff."

I quickly find out why. Each dose is like chugging a full thermos of coffee. My heart races. I start nervously rubbing the back of my neck throughout the day. I pace around in tight little circles while waiting for things to come out of the office printer. My muscles start to feel tight and dense, and I begin compulsively flexing my biceps, not because I want to build them up, but because they just want to *move,* dammit.

But most of all, I've become an emotional creature I can't recognize. I'm sobbing in my car, sobbing in locked bathrooms, sobbing on my couch at home. To be sure, anyone would grieve for lost ears and fear an uncertain future, but *these* feelings are like a jagged slash torn in the beige fabric of my life. Normally I am formal, correct, restrained, the wryly funny analytical type. But the steroids have wrenched me as open as a conch shell.

In Carlos Castaneda's books, don Juan speaks of drugs as teachers: peyote is a guardian and an advisor, and mescaline is the gateway to the other world. Steroids, too, are a teacher. They teach me how to grieve, how to cry, at a time when grief and tears are what I need. Under their brutal influence I begin to write, seizing the opportunity to speak with a raw frankness about my life, my fears, my hearing, and what is about to happen to me. I'm completely deaf, I'm in an eternal cacophony, I'm sobbing every hour on the hour, and I'm pouring out words.

In the *Divine Comedy* Dante speaks of times where "the veil grows thin," where it becomes easy for the traveler to cross the barriers between the earthly and the divine, the seen and the unseen. This is such a time. I am a wreck, but a potently reconstructible one. All that sobbing has made my face go transparent. The shock of total deafness and impending reconstruction has unmoored me from my familiar attitudes and assumptions, breaking me down to first principles, leaving me like a stem cell, embryonic, totipotent. I am emotionally raw, tender with grief and fear, but perceiving the world with such clarity and precision that my former self now seems blind and mundane. The drugs teach me what it is like to be *new.* It is as if the universe is whispering into my now deaf ear, "*Now. Now* is your chance. You have been torn down in body and soul. Go through the change and come out new. *Rebuild.*"

If I want to hear clocks ticking again, people's voices, a lover's murmur, I will have to go through *the change.* The prospect evokes a primitive terror. Before I got my hearing aids I was a mute, fearful little savage, taking in the few words I could grasp with utter literalness. In preschool I was informed that I would become a bird. I took this to mean that I would be changed into an eerie new shape: *wings. beak. eye.* The prospect of this eldritch transformation so terrified me that I came home crying and screaming. Much later I would realize that it was just a metaphor for labeling the kids on the first and second floors (the kids upstairs were the "Birds," those downstairs the "Bears"). But the shaping terrors of childhood never really depart, they only mature into more sophisticated forms. I was going to become a cyborg: *silicon. electrodes. code.*

As a child I had watched wide-eyed as Don Knotts fell into the sea in *The Incredible Mr. Limpet* and was transformed, in a series of agonizing stages, into a fish. Could such things really happen? I wasn't quite sure, but when adults offered to turn me into a bird, the prospect chilled me to the bone. Now I dreamed of computer chips lancing into my head and woke to the realization that the dream was a prediction. The sheer psychic shock of that. The chaos it evoked in the orderly bookshelves of my life.

While the computer would not change me beyond all recognition, it would nevertheless be woven into my body in ways that anyone would find unnerving. There would be a post-surgical scar, which although eventually hidden by re-grown hair would be nonetheless present to my appalled gaze the day after surgery. There would be a tactile bump on my skull a millimeter or two high, obvious to my own fingers and those of a lover's. Most of all, there would be the interface — the plastic *thing* that would stick onto my skull. It would suck itself into place with startling soft firmness, an electromagnetic soul kiss to start the day, and cling there like a remora, odd and obscurely frightening to strangers. Transmitting data generated by complex algorithms with strange acronyms — SPEAK, ACE, CIS, SAS. (Put in that order, they sounded like a strangely intimate telegram from an emotionless intelligence.) The somberly impressive cost: fifty thousand dollars.

And the utter strangeness of the journey. The ritual scarification of surgery, the thirty-day silent period between surgery and activation to let the incision heal, and the crossing into a domain of experience that few people could ever know. Mysterious devices sticking inside and out of my body, crunching numbers like mad. A cyborg. The real thing. Not science fiction. *Me.*

I had long lived a life surrounded by computers, from the TI-83 I had in high school to the successions of computers on my desktop. Now the computer would go *inside* my body, literally woven into my flesh, in my *head.* Running do-loops in a language compiled from C, updating an array of internal variables thirty-two million times a second. I locked myself in my office and cried as I thought of getting a little plastic model of the inner ear and symbolically burying it in my garden. Saying goodbye to the organic ear I used to have, and preparing for its terrifyingly rational reconstruction.

I would not have been so frightened a decade earlier. I used to be uncritically, eagerly in love with computers. In ninth grade my parents bought me a programmable TI calculator, and I spent hours devising programs that would make it play blackjack and tic-tac-toe. Over the years I owned a succession of computers and learned four programming languages. I did my master's in Shakespearean drama because I loved words as well as code, but computers let me build beautiful machines out of ideas, castles in the air held up on delicate struts of logic. For my dissertation I wrote twenty thousand lines of code to create a Web-based program that let students in my literature and composition classes work on projects together outside of the classroom. It worked. It won awards. It got me my Ph.D.

Computers were an elegant, productive addiction — and like all addicts, I began to realize that I was paying a terrible price. In the end, after all those hours at the keyboard, I was still a man sitting alone in a room staring at a computer screen. I had no girlfriend, no family of my own, not even enduringly close friendships apart from the ones I had already developed in high school and college.

My addiction came at least partly from being hard of hearing. I was agonizingly slow to acquire the social graces while growing up. Social norms are not taught, they are overheard, but the one thing even the most skilled deaf people cannot do is overhear. I did not know until high school that people went to parties on the weekends. Community? Intimacy? Like car accidents, they only happened to other people. In my freshman year of college I was so desperate to meet women that in my first month I knocked on *every single door* of the dorm and introduced myself, a memory that still makes me cringe twenty years later. Day after day, I ate alone in the cafeteria at Brown. I had friends, yes, good ones, but just a few, not enough to book all those lunches and dinners. I longed to have a body that didn't need to eat. It was not until I was twenty-five that I had my first girlfriend, and even after that, relationships were few and far between. I was an unbearable teenage nerd, fascinated by computers, miserable with desire, and wholly in love with the idea of the machine. The computer offered me escape and respite, the feeling of control and power.

Computers could connect people, I had argued in my dissertation, and so they could — *if* their use was embedded in a context that was already social and personal, such as the classroom. But absent that, they were machines whose main outputs were logic and loneliness. For me the proof was that my persistent efforts at online dating had met with virtually complete failure: it offered no social context in which I could be judged as a human being. Most online dating sites ask one to specify one's height and the height of one's ideal mate. They also — and here is the rub — enable one to search for people who are only above a given height. I am five-feet-four in my shoes, and it depresses me no end that most women specify, in their profiles, that they want a mate between five-ten and six-two. eHarmony is positively tyrannical about it, matching men *only* with shorter women. As far as the computer is concerned, I am not five-four; I am invisible. The computer utterly rationalizes dating by enabling people to search for potential mates by numerical specifications, eliminating the goofy serendipity of life in a human context.

Because computers are the ultimate expression of abstract logic, they invite the creation of systems that are *only* about logic. That level of abstraction enables programmers to disregard utterly the world of human feelings and needs. All that matters to them is the theoretical beauty of machine logic. The tragedy is that the problems that *cannot* be precisely characterized and neatly solved happen to be the most important ones: communication, understanding, collaboration, negotiation. Love.

As I entered the second half of my thirties I began to feel, as Dante had, that I had lost the path of my life — indeed, that I had never found the path to begin with. I had several close friends scattered around the country, but no one I could just call up and go out for coffee with. I depended on no one, but then again, no one depended on me. Most painfully of all, I found establishing relationships with women nearly impossible. It took me longer to go from puberty to my first relationship (1976–1989) than it took the entire United States government to design and land a spacecraft on the moon (1961–1969). Again and again I made overtures and was rejected. I had always been *sort of:* sort of hearing, sort of socially aware, and as one dating prospect ambiguously said to me, sort of adorable. I felt, as a result, sort of human.

Even as I put the finishing touches on my dissertation, then, I was becoming increasingly disenchanted with computers. They certainly had not met *my* most poignant needs. I frequently reread Frank Herbert's *Dune* trilogy, which is set in a future that has outlawed computers. It doesn't object to technology in general: it embraces spaceships, weaponry, chemistry, and heavy machinery of all kinds. But computers were long ago outlawed during its "Butlerian Jihad," a religious movement that defined the automation of thought as profane. Its battle cry was "Thou shalt not make a machine in the likeness of a man's mind." The need to handle information did not go away, however, so in place of computers are *mentats,* human beings trained to achieve prodigious powers of memorization and data analysis.

Dune's universe focuses on developing human rather than machine powers. Its characters are intensely alive, bursting with inner monologues and ambitions and relationships. Not that I would necessarily want to live in *Dune*'s universe: it's also feudal, violent, autocratic, and totally lacking in what we would call civil liberties. But the gains and the losses apparently couldn't be separated. Take computers away, Herbert seemed to be saying, and what you lost in rationality and orderliness you gained in a human capacity to enter into true relationships with the self and the world. You can have one kind of civilization or the other, *Dune* implied, but not both.

That was why I both loved and hated computers. I loved their pleasures and seductions and conveniences. I hated the hyper-rational, lonely society that their remorseless logic had let human beings so easily create.

And then in Becky's office I was staring at a computer in my palm that was going to go *inside* me. My very body would have technical specifications. Programming language, C. Number of auditory channels, eight. Electrode array refresh rate, either analog or 833 cycles per second, depending on the software. Number of transistors, 140,000. Data transfer rate through the skin, 1.1 million bits per second. Processor speed, 32 million cycles per second. Now the computer would have a grip on me that I would never, ever be able to escape.

I would have to become a cyborg who was deeply suspicious of computers. If I ever chose to embark on a Butlerian Jihad, my first logical target would have to be myself.

The medical system gathers me up into its routine of tests. One of my first stops is the MRI machine, which will peer deep into my skull to see whether surgery is feasible. It's hulking, huge, enormous — a cylindrical superconducting magnet so powerful that it can yank unchained oxygen tanks into its maw from across the room. I am deprived of every piece of metal on my body plus, of course, my wallet with all of its magnetically encoded credit cards. Then I am slid tenderly into the machine's narrow birth canal. The computer may get inside me eventually, but today I am getting inside it.

I lie very still, per instructions. I cannot help eyeballing what little I can see: the off-white curve of the chamber, blankly emitting the confining grandeur of Washington Metro stations; the metal array encircling my head to focus the magnetic field lines; and nothing else whatsoever. I catch myself thinking it would be a nice idea to position a small TV above the patient's head, to fill the lonely forty-five minutes. But it would certainly be destroyed by the magnetic field. Machines can't survive in here. Once I had the implant embedded in my head, I would not be allowed in or even near this room again. In fact, above the MRI's underground chamber is a small outdoor garden whose perimeter is ringed with signs reading sternly: PERSONS WITH PACEMAKERS, NEUROSTIMULATORS, OR METALLIC IMPLANTS MUST NOT ENTER THE LANDSCAPED AREA. Twenty-first-century cherubim and seraphim, banishing me from the Eden of the innocently organic.

The machine grinds, clicks, and hums around me. To my surprise, I feel an artless joy. This is just where I love to be, deep inside elegant machines doing mysterious invisible things at high speed. I am eerily aware that *right now* the computer is probing my head with magnetic fields, executing tens of thousands of lines of code, assembling megabytes of data that will lay bare the inmost contours of my ear. Words like *sagittal, transverse,* and *spline* drift through my mind, although I am only vaguely aware of what they mean. The poetry of technology. Somewhere out of sight, megabytes of data purl onto a server's hard disk.

How was I going to go through *the change?* As a lifelong reader of literature, I already had some answers at hand. A mind richly stocked with stories can select from them as needed, applying narrative to the chaos of experience in order to move ahead with greater sureness to an imagined resolution. When I failed an important exam in grad school, I thought of Odysseus clinging to the fragments of his wrecked ship at sea and remembered that he had still managed to get home to Ithaca. The myth gave me heart and hope.

Now I needed a story not of survival, but of transformation. Pinocchio? Well, not really. Pinocchio was turned into a real live boy as a reward for virtue, and it was done *for* him. Steve Austin? Possibly. But the Steve Austin of the TV show was problematic. To be sure, I had been fascinated by *The Six Million Dollar Man* when it ran in the 1970s. But Steve Austin was a Hollywood cyborg, steely, impassive, and impervious to pain. The nerd in me had loved that image. And yet I could not help feeling skeptical, even then, of the implication that having bionic limbs and organs also entailed having a mechanical soul. Hollywood's depiction of the cyborg seemed like a cheat, a poor bargain: to become more than human, you also had to become less than human. You had to give up your soul to the machine.

But Martin Caidin's novel *Cyborg*, the inspiration for the TV show, had given me an entirely different perspective on Steve Austin. The book version of Steve Austin was resentful, disciplined, and ambitious, a flawed human being who lashed out at his own doctors and engineers yet also collaborated with them in the project of rebuilding himself. More than anything else, Caidin's novel is about Austin's painful transformation and his gradual acceptance of his new body. Acting as Virgil to his Dante is Rudy Wells, his flight surgeon, who guides him with endless patience. At one point

Austin is furious because he continues to fall while running and Wells says to him,

> "You *are* a clumsy kid. Can't you understand that? Biologically, that happens to be the fact. Oh, for God's sake, Steve, you *know* the score. Physiologically, much of your body is that of an adult child. Your system is learning things all over again at superspeed. But it's still *confused.* The problem isn't in the bionics limbs. It's in your own nerve network."

Hollywood cyborgs are often ungainly, but they are not *clumsy.* Clumsiness is a purely human trait. And Steve Austin has a very human reaction to Wells's attempts to explain his own body to him:

> Steve looked at him. "Are you patronizing me, Doc?"
>
> "No, you son of a bitch, I am not."
>
> "Well, you damn well are acting like it!" In a sudden burst of rage he swept the table clean of all objects; ash trays, manuals, coffee cups went crashing to the floor.

It was Caidin's story of struggle and transformation, rather than the ones offered by Hollywood, that served me best twenty-five years later. For me *Cyborg* became a map of the unlighted journey I was about to traverse. Like Steve Austin's, my body would have to build up its own "memory banks" of the new "data feeds" (and they would *literally* be data feeds). I would become an adult child, learning how to hear all over again at superspeed, compressing into days and weeks what takes an infant years to learn.

But I did not yet understand, going in, why Steve Austin was so angry. To be sure, surgery and transformation is a difficult experience, but where did the *rage* come from? Shouldn't he be *excited?* Grateful? Eager to learn and improve? But I would come to understand. Oh, boy, would I be angry. Would I ever.

Yet that was part of the transformation. In acquiring the body of my teenage dreams, I would have the chance to become the adult I wanted to be. To cast off, in my long *agon* with the machine, the longstanding frustrations left over from an unfinished adolescence. To reject the worthless bargain offered by Hollywood, and negotiate a better one. To become a *cyborg*. In real life. On my own terms, in my own way.

2. Surgery

> Mothers in one Central African nation report that on discovering that their child was deaf, their first thought was to verify that their ancestors had been properly buried.
>
> — HARLAN LANE, *The Mask of Benevolence*

AMBULATORY SURGERY, the sign above the front desk says. This surgery is considered straightforward enough for me to ambulate right out of the hospital once the anesthesia wears off. Never mind that the surgeon's whirling drill will pass within one millimeter of my facial nerve, two of my jugular artery, two of my brain. Plug in that circuit board and pack me off home.

Strange how mundane the morning is, on a day where in an hour or so I'm going to be an unconscious body on a table having my head drilled open. It's a fine day, the sun's shining, people are strolling around with thoughts and urgencies in their heads that have absolutely nothing to do with me. There's nothing left to decide or arrange. All I have to do this morning is go wherever people point me.

The lady at the desk hands me a clipboard with a couple of forms. One of them warns me that surgery always entails risks, including infection, paralysis, and death. Yeah, yeah. I scribble my signature on each form and hold out my wrist for the inevitable plastic bracelet.

The waiting room is crowded and quiet. Though it's pleasantly decorated with beige chairs and magazines on Formica tables, it's still a limbo where people await the future with set, private faces. I flip through an antique copy of *Newsweek*. When my dad shows up we sit together, neither of us saying much.

Then I'm called (my dad taps my arm) and I'm admitted to the inner sanctum, a long room with beds separated by cloth dividers. I climb into a bed, feeling a little silly. I'm perfectly healthy: why shouldn't I just walk into the OR? But the logic of this process involves immobilizing me so that I can be controlled. Hospitals are factories where bodies are processed by the clock, and this requires standardizing me so that I can be incorporated into the routine without a fuss. The bed makes me into a unit that can be tracked and injected and wheeled around.

My dad stands by the bed, and Becky shows up to say hello. I'm so excited to see her, I wiggle my toes. She asks me how I am, and I say, "I'm doing good. I'm ready. I'm *very* ready." This thing is the *ultimate* gadget, and I get a whole dramatic and expensive process to go along with it.

The anesthesiologist materializes to put in the IV for the anesthesia. I watch with interest as he numbs the area with a small shot, then puts in the line. There's almost no discomfort, which surprises me because the last time I had an IV I had hated every second of it. But this time it's fine. I say, craning my neck to look back at him, "I don't need any sedative before the operation. I want to be awake to say hello to Dr. Roberson and the team." But Becky motions to him with a thumb and forefinger held together: *just a little.* I glare at her resentfully: *don't you think I'm man enough to handle this?* But it's too late to protest, because a second later *whooo,* my whole body tingles and glows as if someone's just dumped a handful of pixie dust into my brainpan.

Then an orderly shows up at the foot of my bed, there's a *bump* and a jerk, and I'm rolling toward the operating room. Doors bump open in front of me and I'm suddenly surrounded by gleaming surfaces and spiky angles. I'm eager to look around, but I'm not sure what constitutes polite patient behavior, so I settle for a quick gestalt sweep of monitors, green walls, lights, and equipment on racks. A surgical resident appears on my left after I've been transferred to the operating table, and I tell him I've read an article on the surgical technique and so have a pretty good idea of what's about to happen. What I'm really doing is tossing ropes across time to the other side of the operation, trying to bind past and future together across the chasm that awaits. I can feel the bustle and clatter around me as the surgical team spins up to takeoff speed. It is like riding a roller coaster upward to the first great plunge, strapped in and committed. Whatever dazzling truth lies on the other side of that arc is completely unknown. The only thing to do is breathe deeply and wait.

The anesthesiologist puts a clear plastic mask over my mouth. This puzzles me because the anesthesia is intravenous, so I ask, "What's this?" The anesthesiologist pulls down his mask so I can read his lips and says, "Oxygen." *Oh, oxygen,* I think to myself, *breathe deep, pure oxygen's good stuff to have coming into your bloodstream at a time like this.* And then I am in oblivion, beyond time and memory and dreams.

In 1967 the word *deaf* had not yet crystallized in my parents' minds, but they were growing increasingly worried. I ignored them whenever they called to me. At age two and a half I had a vocabulary of perhaps fifteen words, most of which I mispronounced, like *squttit* for *squirrel* (note how it looks the same on the lips).

I remember that time very well. It was a nightmarish dream of my parents moving to and fro, the alternation of day and night, the hypnotic textures of wallpaper and carpets, and the tepid glow of the forty-watt bulb in the hallway after I was put to bed. Most of what I remember is not people or events, but spaces and textures and feelings.

Since I had nothing but vision, the visual impressed itself on me with hallucinatory force. I was inconsolably terrified by the fog rising off the surface of a motel's indoor pool. The pool was inside an inflated canvas dome whose curved surface and khaki color were troubling enough, but the fog rising up from the water made the far end of the pool look vague and indistinct. Space itself looked different over there, turbid and malevolent, and I screamed until my father carried me out. He probably thought I was afraid of falling in the water. Nothing so simple.

And I remember riding on my father's shoulders as he walked down the motel's curving hallway (not that I knew the words *curving, motel,* or *hallway*). My grandfather (not that I knew the word *grandfather*) walked ahead of us with his self-assured, roly-poly gait. As he walked, he stayed in one place. We were moving, yet he was still; the doors were still, yet they glided past us. I absorbed this visual antinomy with such intensity that the scene replayed itself in my dreams, done up in Day-glo colors. I slept and dreamed, only to wake up to a world that was itself a dream.

I was going to a preschool back then, and my main memories of the place are of chilly fear. The sidewalk leading up to it seemed at least five hundred feet long and I walked it with slow reluctant feet, dreading the severe old lady who stood at the entrance each morning and coldly shook my hand as I crossed the transom. Throughout the day I followed the crowd or was steered by the old lady's scaly grip on my shoulders. I made no friends at all, and I have not even the vaguest memory of the faces of the other children.

I was a very peculiar little kid in 1967, so my mother took me to an ear-nose-throat specialist, unloaded her worries, and watched as he rapped tuning forks and peered in my ears. The doctor announced that I looked healthy enough.

"But, Doctor, he's not talking. I call to him and he doesn't even turn around. I don't think he even knows his own name."

"Well, *my* daughter didn't talk until she was four years old. Kids develop at different rates. Just you wait, he'll start talking when he's good and ready."

My mother didn't know what to say to this. At twenty-four, she was too young and inexperienced to mount much of a defense against medical avuncularity. And one didn't question doctors in those days. But still . . . something just wasn't right. She had had a chilly, tight feeling in the pit of her stomach for weeks.

"Doctor . . . when I call his name, *he doesn't even turn around.*"

The doctor's voice took on a patronizing tone. He might as well have said out loud, *Another neurotic mother.* "Tell you what. If you would like to get his hearing tested, I'll give you a referral."

Which he did. My mom towed me home, feeling both relieved and confused, and smarting from the tone of the doctor's voice. When my dad came home from work, the conversation was straightforward.

"The doctor says there's nothing wrong with his hearing."

My dad looked over at me and said slowly, "Yes, there is."

On a hot day in June 1967 my parents took me to an audiologist at Queens College in New York City. As I sat in a soundproofed booth on my mom's lap, he ran me through a series of tones that became progressively louder. I just looked at him and then around the room. Nothing interesting here.

The audiologist finished the test, spent a few minutes drawing what looked like a line graph, then broke the news: I had, at the very least, a severe hearing impairment. I could hear loud sounds, but not speech. In short, functionally speaking, I was deaf.

My mother sums up their day following this news with the word *brainlock.* In brainlock they got up, paid for the visit in cash, took the bus to my grandparents' home nearby (I looked around at the traffic with great interest), and the minute the door closed behind them, burst into horrified tears. *Deaf. Our son is deaf.*

How could a doctor, or my parents for that matter, miss the fact that I was deaf? Unfortunately, deafness can be subtle and difficult to diagnose. It looks a lot like mental retardation, for example. My hearing was good enough for me to hear concussive sounds, so the homegrown test of bang-something-behind-the-kid would often cause me to turn around. What I couldn't hear was *speech.*

The very first thing my parents did upon bringing me home was sit me in front of the TV and position my ear directly against the speaker. It was then that my parents at last knew deep down that I was deaf, for my face lit up in a delighted *wow, what's this?* reaction. In that instant, their whole understanding of the past changed. Now they knew that to me the TV had been nothing more than small, flat people moving around at random. All those conversations at the dinner table — silent movies. It hit my dad in a rush that in three years, the only times I had ever heard his voice had been when I was in his lap.

In the dictionary, the word *deaf* follows the word *dead:* dead air, deadbeat, deadwood . . . deaf. For parents, a child's handicap often causes a grieving not incomparable to that following death. Every parent prayerfully imagines their child's first steps, bat mitzvah or first communion, first date, graduation, marriage, and beyond, and their hopes range ever forward into that vague future in which they find their own grave but not their child's. But when their child cannot see, or hear, or walk, those multifold futures die. They can no longer see their child as a strong, confident, proud adult. In its place they see nightmare images of wheelchairs, white canes, hearing aids, halting speech, and lifelong dependency. My mother and father walked around for days in sick horror.

But if one has to be born deaf, it helps to have formidably educated parents. My mother had majored in, of all things, special education for the blind; my father was (as he still is) a child psychologist. They set to work identifying specialists, technologies, and options. Sign language was considered and relegated to a final option, to be deployed only if all else failed. They wanted to see if I could be integrated into normal life, speaking English and having the opportunities available to people who could speak and hear.

The next move, then, was to see what hearing aids could do for me. For that, my parents took me to the League for the Hard of Hearing in New York, where an audiologist named Judy Lambert put my ears through a full workup and recommended aids made by a company named Radioear. The very name makes me laugh today, harking back to a time when radio was invoked as a glorious leading-edge technology. Ironically, it still is; a cochlear implant transmits the signal through the skin by . . . radio. But at the time

"Radioear" meant classic behind-the-ear hearing aids, sitting atop my ears like cats draped over the back of a La-Z-Boy.

Strangely enough, I have no recollection of the day when they were plugged into my ears and turned on for the first time. One would think I'd remember hearing my own voice for the first time, but the memory is gone, perhaps being so novel that my brain had no idea what to do with the experience.

But simply having some hearing was not enough to solve my problems. Linguistically, I was three years behind other children my age, which was a serious problem given that I was four years old. And time was running out fast. If a child gets to the age of four without having acquired fluent and natural diction, chances are slim that he or she ever will. Therefore my parents undertook a crash program to cram three years' worth of language development into me in, oh, about six months.

But how to do that? Judy Lambert referred my parents to the John Tracy Clinic in Los Angeles, founded in 1942 by Spencer Tracy, the actor, and his wife, Louise, after their child John was born deaf. My mom wrote them a letter from New Jersey saying *help!* and promptly got a letter back with the first lesson of a correspondence course in how to educate young deaf children. This course proved to be, in my mom's words, "a lifeline." She'd work with me using the lesson as a guide, and then send notes on my progress to the clinic. In due time a letter would come back with the next lesson, with directions on how to use it to give me the most benefit. These were not off-the-cuff tips; they were pages-long, typed letters responding to what my parents had written and giving detailed instructions on what to do next. The letters gave them the guidance and encouragement they needed to get through the perplexities of raising a deaf child. It was personalized instruction and mentorship of extraordinary quality. Moreover, it was free of charge, supported by the Tracy family's trust fund and various donors.

Now, decades later, the John Tracy Clinic still exists, as does its correspondence course. Much has changed, of course; the clinic now has a Web site, the lessons are now supplemented by videos, and the course texts are available in twenty-three languages. But the course is *still* free, *still* first-rate. Spencer Tracy died in June 1967, right about when the first letters from L.A. were arriving in the mail. To most people his legacy is his film career, but to me, the legacy of him and his wife is *me*. I see him now and then in old movies, and I mentally tip my hat and say, *Thanks, man.*

Based on the lessons arriving periodically in the mail, my mom did things like cutting out pictures from magazines and sorting them into envelopes labeled by letter: apples went into the *A* envelope, boys into the *B* envelope, and so forth. At the kitchen table, I'd pick out a letter I liked and we'd go through the pictures, saying the words together.

My dad tackled my reading development, on the theory that although my ears were shot, my eyes worked just fine. He bought me a box of beige cards, each of which had a picture on one side and a word on the other (see figure 1).

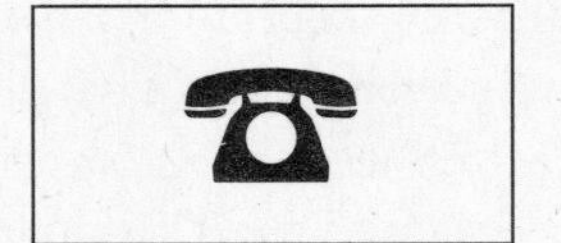

Figure 1

His idea was that words could be treated as ideograms holding meaning purely on their visual properties. This was not Tracy Clinic doctrine; it was my dad's supplement to it. In effect, he cut sound out of the reading loop and taught me printed English as if it were Chinese. This method is now unpopular because success in reading has been strongly linked to how well children can reproduce and manipulate the basic sounds of language — *phonological awareness*, it's called. So few reading teachers would try to do this today.

But it worked for me. Either my father's theory had more to recommend it than current wisdom allows, or I was getting enough input in various other ways that I couldn't help but put things together. Once I had mastered some vocabulary, my dad moved on to syntax, putting cards together in strings to form sentences. *The telephone is white.* I'd nod, because I knew the kitchen phone was white. *The telephone is blue.* I'd shake my head. *The white is telephone.* Oh, Dad, that's painful. Don't *do* that to me. I'd wrinkle my nose and rearrange the cards, already a fussy four-year-old editor.

I loved it. I was born to swim in words. My parents tell me that in the mornings I would pad to the kitchen in my one-piece jammies, drag a chair over to the counter, stand on it so I could appropriate the box of cards, and bring it to them in their bed, asking to go over the words *one more time*, please.

While all this was going on, my mom took me to the local preschool for deaf children for an evaluation. Sure, I was deaf, but was I deaf enough? Would they take me in? The school's president scanned my audiogram with an expert eye, inspected my hearing aids, then took me around the classrooms for the grand tour. Or my mother thought it was a tour; what they were in fact doing was putting me through an informal developmental evaluation. How alert was I to sound? What was my linguistic age? How did I interact with toys? I'm sure I picked up the cardboard bricks and peered through the magnifying glasses: oh, this stuff is interesting. My mom sweated it out. They just *had* to take me. Just *had* to.

I started at Summit Speech School in the spring of 1969, with wobbly hearing aids perched on my small ears. These — plus the constant training I was now getting each day at school and at home — transformed me so fast that today it takes my breath away to think of it. "It was like turning on a light bulb," my mom says. All of a sudden, I was learning dozens of words a week and figuring out the syntax that transformed words into meanings.

So for me, 1967 and 1969 took place in different universes. In 1967 I was a mute, fearful little animal. In 1969 I wore long-sleeved plaid polyester shirts, which I liked, and had a chipped front tooth, which I didn't. Released from the car in front of the school, I'd launch myself down the sidewalk at a run, bound up the front stairs, zip past the elderly receptionist smiling benignly at me from her desk, and (this was the fun part) dash up and down the little two-step ziggurat of stairs that fronted the stairway to the second floor. A flying bank to the right took me through the kitchen, which seemed small even to my pint-sized self, and into the rear classroom. This was where Mrs. Widman (invariably called "Mrs. Woman") and my friends Sam, Bobby, Chris, Mary, and Carl would be.

We were all there, of course, because we were deaf, and generally we were deaf for the same reason. An epidemic of a minor disease, rubella, had passed through the United States between 1962 and 1965. It had caused fevers, joint pain, and rashes in twelve and a half million people. In children and adults, the virus was relatively benign; most people shrugged it off in a few days. But in pregnant women it crossed the placental barrier and homed in on cells in the growing cochlea with grim efficiency.

The six of us in Mrs. Widman's morning class belonged to the "rubella bulge," a cohort of twenty thousand deaf children making their way through the school system *en bloc.* Whenever I meet hearing-impaired people who are not elderly, the odds are very good that they will be my own age. In 1969 a vaccine would be distributed nationwide, making the 1962–1965 rubella epidemic the last one in U.S. history. Too late, of course, for us.

But by now, with my language abilities growing geometrically, the world became a place full of meanings. With my classmates I finger-painted, built houses with the large red cardboard bricks, and peered at various sticky little hands, including my own, through the magnifying glasses. During the game "Button, button, who's got the button?" I knew perfectly well that Mrs. Widman was going to drop a button, secretly, into one of our cupped hands. I finger-painted a car in blue, a drawing of our new Ford LTD station wagon with the most awesomely cool closing headlight covers. Waiting to be picked up at the end of the school day, I would find an oak seed in the yard, break its green whirlybird wings in half, and paste the sap-sticky center on my nose so that I could be a rhinoceros. But I was not a rhinoceros. Finally, I was becoming human.

* * *

And now I am becoming something else: not *in*human, not *post*-human, but *differently* human. My surgeon, Dr. Roberson, shows up around 8:30. At forty-one, he is a solidly built, red-haired man with the sort of open, robust face that young children would like. Were there ever a Butlerian Jihad, he could probably melt into his native North Carolina backwoods and pass himself off as a soft-spoken farmer until he slipped and blurted out a phrase such as "CO_2 laser stapedotomy" in polite company. He has the tall man's courteous habit of bending down just slightly in conversation to bring his face closer to your own. He also shakes hands carefully, curving his arm and cupping his hand so that only the edges of it touch your own, which has the effect of letting you sense both his physical strength and the fact that he holds it in careful reserve.

The anesthesiologist has draped my head and upper body in sterile cloth, so that in a few minutes I have entirely disappeared from view as a human being.* Only my ear and a few inches of scalp are visible through a square in the cloth. I am now deep underwater, frozen, dreamless, taken out of time altogether. I am sustained by machines and an anesthesiologist who monitors numbers on a computer screen rather than watching my face.

At about 9:00 the surgery begins. In seconds, Dr. Roberson slices a two-and-a-half-inch incision behind my ear. That enables him to lift my entire outer ear upward to expose my skull. The nurse rolls the operating microscope into place. About six feet high, it looks bizarrely expressive, like a high-tech dinosaur poised to spring. Since the inner ear is a very small operating area, smaller than a thimble, Dr. Roberson will perform most of the operation while peering through its lenses.

Then he picks up a diamond-studded drill bit. He presses a foot panel and it instantly goes from a dull matte to the color of quicksilver, spinning 85,000 times per second. That's so fast that wherever he puts it, bone simply *isn't* anymore. It flashes into a fog of micron-sized particles. Moving the drill in quick, short strokes, he

* The details from here forward come from an operation I observed seven months later.

begins excavating a tunnel in my mastoid bone toward my cochlea, which is buried an inch and a half deep inside my skull. The reason he goes through my skull rather than my ear canal is that the ear canal is, well, open. There's nothing to which the electrode array can be securely fastened, and puncturing my eardrum would leave the middle ear exposed to the outside world. So he drills toward my cochlea from above and behind my ear, breaking into the house through the back door, so to speak.

But this is an extremely delicate break-in. Right now Dr. Roberson is doing skull base surgery, a specialized field. The base of the skull is a concentrated and complex area with dozens of blood vessels and nerves. Neurosurgeons often call on skull base surgeons just to get them through the area so they can operate on the brain. But this is not brain surgery, not today. Dr. Roberson's drill will travel within millimeters of my brain, but his target is my inner ear, not my cortex.

In about twenty-five minutes the air cavity of my middle ear comes into view, exposing my cochlea. Dr. Roberson puts down the drill and pokes some gel foam into the tunnel to keep bone dust out of it. He raises the microscope away from my head. The first stage of the operation is over.

Then he turns his attention to sculpting a depression behind my ear where the body of the implant will go. This part of the operation is pure carpentry: all he needs to do is create a well just deep enough so that the implant — about an inch square and the thickness of three quarters — will countersink neatly into my skull, creating only the slightest bulge under my skin. The company has helpfully supplied a metal template the size of the casing, and he uses it to check that the hollow is the right size and shape.

While Dr. Roberson has been sculpting the implant bed, the head nurse has been preparing the implant itself. She has torn open a corner of its plastic packaging and poured distilled water into it to protect it from static electricity. That done, she takes it out of the package with tweezers and hands it to Dr. Roberson, who places it on a pad and sets it under the microscope for inspection. The electrode array leaps into sharp and enormously magnified focus on the video screens. It is curiously hard to see clearly: the metal electrodes glitter, throwing off sparks of light, and the silicone surrounding them makes it hard to see where they are. He turns it this way and that, examining the electrode array from various angles. Seen under a microscope, the electrodes are slightly irregular in size and not perfectly evenly spaced. It doesn't have the arrogant regularity of a machine-stamped artifact. That's because it's made by hand by some laboring technician in a clean room in Southern California. (See figures 2 and 3.)

Satisfied with the implant, Dr. Roberson proceeds to fit it into my skull. It snaps in firmly, and he anchors it with metallic sutures threaded through holes he has drilled in the bone on either side of it. Now it is time to insert the electrode array into my cochlea. This is the climax of the operation: it is the moment when the computer is aligned directly against my nerve endings.

But how to get it *in* there? The cochlea is a tight 2¾-rotation spiral where every millimeter entails a turn in direction. How does one insert a wire into a spiral without scraping crudely along the inside, causing cellular havoc equivalent to dragging a ladder against the walls of an art gallery? This was a major problem in the early days of cochlear implant research. Even though the hair cells are shot, the surgeon wants to do as little damage as possible to the auditory nerves and the balance system, which are as crucial as ever. Early trials showed that the act of insertion could do grievous damage; in fact, sometimes the electrodes cut through the delicate internal membranes like a knife. "It cannot . . . simply be pushed into the cochlear spiral as if it were a plumber's snake passing through a curved drainpipe," wrote one scientist ruefully in 1985. Varying the flexibility of the material only exchanged one problem for another. When it was too stiff it couldn't be inserted without damage, but when it was too soft it couldn't be inserted at all.

The problem preoccupied researchers for years until Graeme

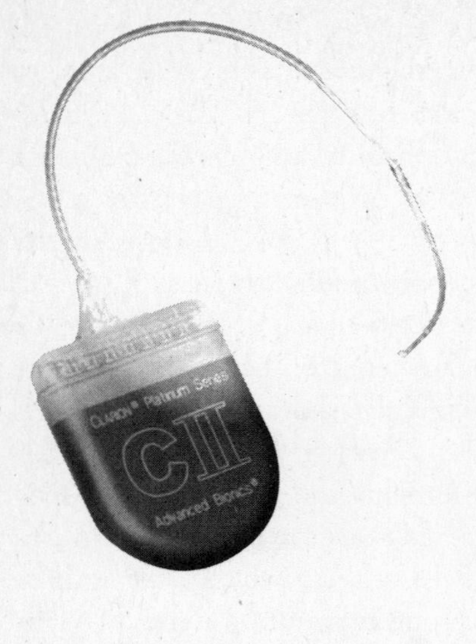

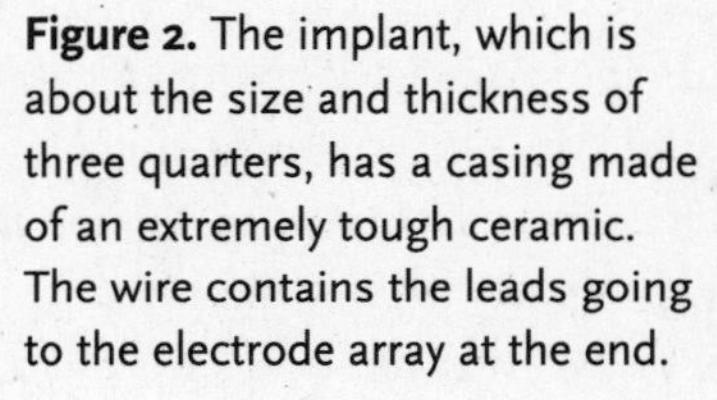

Figure 2. The implant, which is about the size and thickness of three quarters, has a casing made of an extremely tough ceramic. The wire contains the leads going to the electrode array at the end.

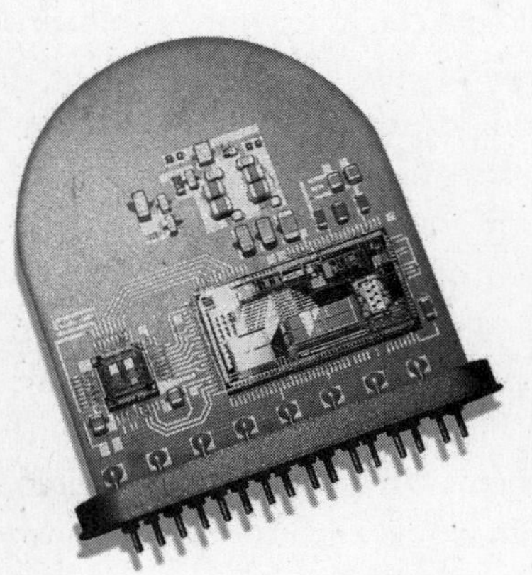

Figure 3. The circuit board inside the implant contains a large chip that processes the incoming radio signal and controls the electrode array, and a small chip that does the hardcore math (about one million operations per second). The other side of the circuit board contains the AM radio antenna, the FM radio transmitter, and the magnet to which the headpiece sticks. Each of the sixteen pins controls one of the electrodes.

Clark, the lead surgeon in developing the Australian version of the implant in the mid-1970s, had a brainstorm. One day, when he was at the beach in Australia, he picked up a spiral-shaped shell and idly began poking grass stems into it, working the problem in his mind. After a while, he discovered that certain kinds of grass, which were stiff at the stem but flexible at the tip, slid smoothly into the shell without so much as cracking. That was it! *Differential stiffness!*

If the electrode array became increasingly stiffer down its length, the flexible tip would lead the way, enabling the rest of the array to obediently follow it around the curve.

Our civilization's greatest accomplishments are built on a tiny scale. The electrode array, less than an inch long, is the product of forty years of research and development. Now Dr. Roberson inserts it in a single smooth motion, using a device that looks a little bit like a syringe. By design, it will penetrate only as far as one and a half rotations; it can't be pushed further than that without risk of damage. Besides, decades of research have shown that this depth is sufficient. The goal is to stimulate the nerves in the *center* of the cochlea, and surrounding it once and then some is all that is needed.

It's done. All that is left to do is back out of the operating area and close up the incision — and then boot the thing up for a minute to make sure it works. Becky comes into the OR, holding a laptop up high so as not to bump it into anything. It runs the software that interfaces with the implant. A month from now, she will use it to activate me. Today, however, all she wants to do is send a telemetric inquiry through my skin to ask it, *Are all sixteen of your electrodes still working?*

In *Cyborg*, Martin Caidin foresaw this moment a quarter-century earlier while writing about Steve Austin's many surgeries, culminating in the one where his new legs were joined to his body:

> Human and human-made were brought together, connected, spliced, wired, sealed. Raw flesh was treated and joined with what was not flesh so that the two might function together as the human entity had performed before the limbs were mutilated and severed.
>
> As he slept, he came back to life. As he swam deep in blackness, electrical probes were applied to his system. His body twisted, his body snapped, as the men attending him worked with feverish anticipation and brooding concern.

While this operation has not been quite so brutal as all that, and the "feverish anticipation and brooding concern" have given way to brisk professionalism in this age of commercialized bionics, my consciousness *has* been obliterated, a surgeon *has* taken a knife to my body, and electronics *have* been fused to my flesh. And now electrical probes will be applied to test that they work as I sleep.

Becky sets the laptop down on a table and runs a serial cable from it to the aluminum-gray box of the processor. Dr. Roberson pulls a white plastic drape over my head and points wordlessly to where the implant is. Becky applies the headpiece and moves it around a little bit until it magnetically tugs itself into place. She turns to the laptop and presses one of the keys on its keyboard, watching its screen. One by one, the software sends pulses of electricity to the electrodes, verifying that each is still responding an inch and a half deep in my skull. In less than a minute she nods briefly to Dr. Roberson. Sixteen for sixteen. It's working.

The field of my ear must lie fallow before its rebirth. When the remaining hair cells died on July 7, 2001, I stumbled and fell, crippled. Now that the computer is in place almost everything in my biological ear — outer ear, ear canal, eardrum, stapes, ossicles, round window, basilar membrane — has been bypassed and rendered irrelevant. Theories vary on whether the surgery will kill off any hair cells that might still be intact, but it hardly matters. I am now totally committed to the computer.

My dad leans over me. I can barely see him without my glasses. The purple turban wrapped around my head feels bulky and strange.

"How are you doing?"

I think about that. Can I *feel* the computer in my skull? Can I feel the electrodes spiraled around my ganglial nerves, metal against flesh, gripping it tight?

I'm not sure if I can actually feel it. But it's got to be in there.

I say weakly, "When I finish booting up Windows 98, Dad, I'll let you know."

The joke falls completely flat. He just gapes at me, confused.

3. Between Two Worlds

> Nothing of him that doth fade,
> But doth suffer a sea-change
> Into something rich and strange.
>
> — SHAKESPEARE, *The Tempest*

IT'S A DAY or two after surgery. I'm home and the purple turban has come off, leaving just a paper bandage behind my left ear. The anesthesia has left me with a walloping hangover. I'm tired, bleary, restless.

I can feel the compact bulk of the implant in my skull. It is strange to think that by now its two computer chips will have warmed up to exactly the temperature of my body, and that they will *stay* at that temperature. I also have the odd feeling that there is a piece of string stuck deep in my ear. Am I actually feeling the wire running to the electrode array? I've sent an e-mail to one of the doctors and he says I'm just feeling fluid draining into my middle ear, but I'm not so sure.

Whatever exactly I'm feeling, there is most definitely something new in my body, something not called for in the original specifications. Dr. Roberson has told me it's fine to sleep on the implanted side, but I'm sure as hell not doing that. What if the weight of my head pushes on the casing and makes the electrode array move around?

Anesthesia does things to your mind. As I'm lying in bed I can visualize with utter clarity the exact, mute shape of the thing, its rounded body, its long electrical lead curled up scorpionlike deep inside my head. If it grew some legs it would look exactly like a bug. A *bug!* I'm seized with a horrible vision of it slashing through my skin and scrabbling out of my head, running hell-bent down the back of my neck on insanely quick little legs. Dragging the electrode array behind it like a silver tail. Tickling obscenely as it skitters over my skin, its ravening mind calculating at 32 megahertz where to go next. Images flash through my head of me holding it up at arm's length while staring at its wriggling legs in sheer horror.

I'm not even dreaming, and I've managed to scare the daylights out of myself. I angle my right arm around my head and run my fingers carefully over where I think the implant is. I can visualize all too clearly a red-rimmed, loose-lipped rip in my scalp with bright rivulets of blood beginning to seep into my hair.

But it's okay. The area feels the same. It's still in there.

I roll over in bed and look at my cat, Elvis, who has picked up his little head and is staring at me. I sit up and drag him into my lap. It's time for an emergency cuddle. I slowly rub my nose in the fur between his ears.

The word *cyborg* is often applied to anyone with an artificial body part, but that's just plain wrong. A person with an artificial hip is not a cyborg, because the hip doesn't make choices about what to do; it just provides mechanical support. Same for artificial teeth, corneas, and knees. They're triumphs of materials science and surgical technique, but they're not cyborg technologies. The essence of cyborgness is the presence of software that makes if-then-else decisions and acts on the body to carry them out.

It is the "acts" part that is important. Even having silicon chips in the body doesn't by itself make one a cyborg. In one of the more egregious misuses of the word, *Time* published an article in 2002 with the tagline, "Jeffrey, Leslie, and their boy Derek will be America's first cyborg family. Are you ready to 'Get Chipped'?" The technology consisted of chips implanted in their forearms containing a little RAM and a radio transmitter — the same technology already implanted in countless dogs and cats across the country. Its function was to announce their presence to light switches, doors, and so forth. The chips were inside their bodies, to be sure, but no control was exerted over their bodies' functioning. They would work just as well embedded in a badge.

On the other hand, a real cyborg technology exerts control of some kind over the body. A pacemaker is a cyborg technology, because it steps in to regulate heart function when it senses defibrillation. This kind of control gets at the heart, so to speak, of what it means to be a cyborg: to have *cybernetic*, meaning "algorithmic and automated," control of the *organism*.

But pacemakers and cochlear implants are very different kinds of cyborg technologies. A pacemaker regulates the pump that keeps your body going, and as long as it works, your life is what it was before. You can forget about it (although I don't doubt that people with pacemakers may be profoundly affected by the knowledge that their life is dependent on a computer). When the control is over your *senses*, however, you can never forget about it. You are living in a new version of reality.

Cultural theorists often claim that in this day and age, *everyone* is a cyborg — that technological society has worked its will on all of us. Chris Hables Gray, in his book *Cyborg Citizen*, writes, "If you have been technologically modified in any significant way, from an implanted pacemaker to a vaccination that reprogrammed your immune system, then you are definitely a cyborg." But this definition is so broad as to be useless. If everyone is a cyborg then no one is; the word loses all definitional power. Using vaccinations as an example is also technically wrong, because vaccinations trigger the immune system only to do what it does normally. Despite his use of the word *reprogrammed*, antibodies exert no ongoing algorithmic control over the body.

Still, many theorists have taken tool use to an extreme and called themselves cyborgs. Steve Mann, a professor at the University of Toronto, has become well-known for developing and wearing portable computer technology that he uses to mediate his perception of reality. All day long he wears a portable computer with a tiny video monitor positioned in front of his right eye. In his book *Cyborg: Digital Destiny and Human Possibility in the Age of the Wearable Computer,* he describes what his system can do. It lets him do e-mail and access the Web. It can function as a video camera, enabling him to take footage of whatever he happens to be looking at. Most significantly, it can mediate his view of what he is looking at by altering the video stream in real time before it reaches his eye. He writes of possibilities such as having the computer blank out billboards (thus eliminating corporate intrusions on one's consciousness) and display messages when a certain object comes into view, such as a message from your spouse reminding you to pick up milk when a milk carton comes into view.

But is Steve Mann truly a cyborg, as he calls himself? I would argue that he is not, because while his technologies provide his body with information, they do not cybernetically control it. In his book *Redesigning Humans,* Gregory Stock offers a more precise term for people like Steve Mann: *fyborg,* or "functional cyborg." The difference is that fyborgs are augmented by externally worn equipment, whereas cyborgs are physically fused with the equipment. "Most people with a hearing problem, for instance, have a fyborgian hearing aid," Stock writes, "rather than a cyborgian cochlear implant."

In fact, the word *fyborg* describes virtually all human beings, whereas the word *cyborg* describes only a few. Our bodies have been augmented by technology for thousands of years: plows, shovels, flint knives, quill pens. To point to constant technology use as evidence that the user is a "cyborg" is an empty claim. It's just a glamorous way of saying that human beings are tool-users.

Other theorists, such as Donna Haraway, use the word *cyborg* more metaphorically to name the psychological and social condition of being an assemblage of multiple and conflicting perspectives. Much as Robocop, a human policeman shot up by bad guys and restored with mechanical parts, experiences the universe differently in his new body, all human beings have multivalent and constructed viewpoints. For Haraway, all human beings are cyborgs in a personal and political sense.

There are important insights that can come from this perspective, but in the end the word *cyborg* does relatively little work here, too. It's just a glamorous way of saying that people are complex, fragmented, and contradictory.

To be meaningful and useful, then, the word *cyborg* has to do something new. It has to name a kind of relationship with technology that has not existed before. Mediating a person's perception of reality by computationally controlling nerve endings inside the body is most definitely new. Glasses don't do that; cell phones don't do that; even pacemakers and artificial hips don't do that. But a cochlear implant does.

Midpoint. I am now twelve days post-op, twelve days pre-activation. The implant has not yet been booted up, so I am as deaf as ever. Twelve more days of healing need to pass before Becky gives me the processor that will bring it to life with tiny bursts of electricity.

So much has changed: in my life, in my attitudes, and in the world. September 11 took place five days after my surgery and split the nation's history into Before and After. I am in shock like everyone else, groping for my bearings politically as well as physically. I saw the towers fall in a dreamlike silence.

With a hearing aid in my still-organic right ear I have maybe 5 percent of the hearing of a normal person. Yet I have become better and better at making use of the thin trickle of information I do get. All I can hear with my eyes closed is the equivalent of vibrations. I can detect the presence of voices, but not understand them. Yet with my eyes open, I can have reasonably successful conversations with many people. Together, lip-reading plus a little bit of sound information often gets the message across. How much bandwidth can a human being lose and still remain connected to his fellows? For me, the answer would be: nearly all of it.

My situation is not unlike that of the Galileo spacecraft, which was crippled when its main antenna failed to open en route to Jupiter. Its data transfer rate dropped from 134,000 bits per second down to the 16 bits per second that its secondary antenna could transmit. But its engineers were able to reprogram the spacecraft in flight with data-compression algorithms so that the secondary antenna could transmit 120 bits per second. That's far less than 134,000, of course, but it was a brilliant hack that enabled the mission to achieve many of its goals nonetheless.

I have executed my own internal hacks by evolving entirely new ways to have conversations with people. It stuns me how far I have come since the day I went deaf, when I had to have people write down every word for me. Now, I can have conversations that are fairly close to normal. When I begin a conversation, I experience a moment of "priming" as I power myself up to full alertness. I can almost feel my brain humming as it starts soaking up extra glucose and oxygen, getting ready. I swivel to look my interlocutor directly in the eye. My head lowers slightly. I lock on.

When my conversation partner talks, I am depending almost equally on lip-reading and hearing. One modality resolves ambiguities in the other. I realized, very early on, that my conversation partners needed considerable reassurance from me that I was in fact understanding them. In a sense they were flying blind, not knowing what I was hearing. I evolved a technique of rapidly repeating key fragments of their speech back to them as a form of protocol checking.

On a fine mid-afternoon I'm having a late lunch with Kristin, who works down the hall from me. Today I want to hear — well, sort of hear — what she's been up to.

She says, "Well, I'm doing work for the Carnegie Corporation —"

"Carnegie Corporation," I say, *sotto voce,* nodding.

"— it's a project to study how teachers learn to teach in alternative certification programs —"

"Alternative certification —"

"— and see if we can figure out what makes those programs more or less effective in preparing teachers."

It's time for me to give her a paraphrase. "You figure out the success factors for teachers in alternative certification programs."

She nods, confirming. "And I'm also doing some work for the . . . ates physician in techniques where arbpurm errum isn't . . ."

I cock my head. "A black physician." Given the subject matter, I know this is probably not what she said. I'm giving her my nearest match, so she can see where things went off the rails.

She repeats the phrase. "The Bates Physician."

No, that can't be it either. I cock my head ever so slightly toward the notepad. Kristin's hand is already moving there. She writes a *G*, an *a*, and a *t*. Her hand is going on to the next letter, but I've seen all I need.

"The Gates Foundation," I say, crisply.

"Right. For the Gates Foundation, I'm —"

It's like juggling, where she tosses me a great many words and I artfully toss back the critical ones, slipping them into the sidestream of our conversation. A crippled spacecraft, substituting smarts for speed. Data compression and verification. Protocol checking. Handshaking. *Yes, your message got through, keep going.*

But I am also getting messages from what I can only assume is my subconscious. Auditory hallucinations are common in people who suddenly go deaf. Most of them are musical; researchers have solemnly tabulated what various people hear, including *Auld Lang Syne, Pomp and Circumstance, Danny Boy, Yellow Rose of Texas,* and (this delights me, as it is HAL's dying song) *Daisy.*

I get music like *Atmospheres,* but I also get poetry. As I write this, a line from Ezra Pound's *Cantos* is repeating itself obsessively in the private soundbox of my head:

Pull down thy vanity,
Paquin pull down!

It repeats itself over and over again, hollow and breathy yet resonant, like a chant emanating from a cave, or from a thousand spirits of the underworld who don't really care about being in sync. The consonants are drawn out, and the short *a* in *Paquin* is louder and sharper than the rest of the line. My auditory experience, then, is like this:

Pullllll down thy vanity,
  PAquin . . . pull downnnnnnn!
Pullllll down thy vanity,
  PAquin . . . pull downnnnnnn!
Pullllll down thy vanity,
  PAquin . . . pull downnnnnnn!
Pullllll down thy vanity,
  PAquin . . . pull downnnnnnn!

I time it: each cycle takes five full, round seconds. That comes out to twelve per minute, 720 per hour. It's gone on for about three hours. That's 2,160 repetitions so far.

Fortunately, I seem to be able to bear it. It's like moving into an apartment above a busy street in Manhattan. The din! The roar! But after a while, one learns to tune it out and pay attention to other things.

What I want to know is, out of the thousands of lines of English poetry I've read in my life, why am I getting *this* line? The simplest theory is that because the words are round, resonant, and rhythmic, they match the subjective frequencies and tempos of my tinnitus. To put it another way, my mind currently finds them to be the most meaningful interpretation of the random noise in my inner ear.

But still. English poetry is full of round, resonant, rhythmic lines. Why this one? I look up the line in context:

What thou lovest well is thy true heritage
What thou lov'st well shall not be reft from thee . . .

Learn of the green world what can be thy place
In scaled invention or true artistry,
Pull down thy vanity,
  Paquin pull down!

Ezra Pound wrote these lines in clear-eyed grief and humility, while he was in prison awaiting trial for treason (during World War II he had made radio broadcasts supporting Mussolini, whom he had admired). "Paquin" was a Parisian dressmaker renowned for showy clothing, so for Pound he symbolizes vanity.

Over the next two years this fragment of poetry would come to mean different things to me. On this day it is about "pulling down," of being broken and rebuilt. Using what artistry I can to learn of my place in the green world.

And what will it be like? To be *activated*?

People offer me words like *robotic* and *artificial* to describe the sound, but such words are just labels, as divorced from experience as the word *green* is from the sensation of seeing green. Becky cautions me that everyone's experience is different. I will simply have to find out for myself.

I can vaguely guess at the strangeness of it, though. Imagine that you have been very nearsighted all your life, but still able to recognize faces, get around, even drive. Suddenly your vision fails and all you can see are vague shadows. Surgeons insert expensive machinery behind your irises. Three days follow, in a fog. Your eyes hurt. The fog lifts and you feel better, but must wait a month while the incisions heal. Then you go back to the clinic, still stumbling in blindness, to have this alien new part of your body turned on. And then you see again, not sharper, necessarily, but more, and brighter, and — is that what red looks like? That is green, yes? Matching up your old world with your new one. And sometimes there is no available match. Your friend's face looks more detailed when you use this particular software, but has better color with that software. Which is better? More useful? More enjoyable? Snowshoeing through a storm of data, sifting for the familiar, making sense of the unfamiliar. Living in a different body, learning what it gives you.

In the meantime, life continues. My Palm Pilot slowly fills up with appointments and social events for after Activation Day. Entering those events feels strange, like knowing I'm going to show up female instead of male, or Catholic instead of Jewish. *Wings. beak. eye.* I'm tossing ropes across a chasm I can't see. Trusting that they're going to anchor somewhere on the other side.

4. Activation

"We'll find out soon enough, Art," Steve told him. He didn't like the sudden turn of conversation. He would be activated, which was a hell of a word to use about a human, and yet it was the only word that applied. He'd be activated and they'd find out if theory would work.

— MARTIN CAIDIN, *Cyborg*

OCTOBER 1, 2001. Today, I will walk into the California Ear Institute a deaf man; I will walk out a hearing one. In biblical times making the deaf hear was a sign of godhood because only a god could do it. In the twenty-first century, human beings do it routinely, but the idea still evokes a shivery awe. It *does* seem miraculous. Unlike body parts such as legs or hearts, the sensory organs are hard to understand in naive mechanical terms, so restoring them seems perilously akin to magic. The leg is a lever, the heart is a hydraulic pump. But the eyes and ears are passageways of the soul.

In the morning I move slowly and carefully in picking up forks and tying my shoes, conserving every calorie for what lies ahead. Often my breath catches and my stomach tightens as I exhale, for I'm on the edge of tears. In my mind is an image of me reaching out to touch a massive stone door that will wheel open to reveal a blinding light.

At the Institute Becky arrives late, the morning's surgery having gone overtime. With her is Cache, a round-faced audiologist from Wyoming who, I will later discover, is constantly switching from one permutation of facial hair to another. He's new to the center, and I am the very first patient he will have observed all the way from surgery to activation.

The exertion from the small talk I've made with my friends Margaret and Paula, who have come along to lend support, has left me tired and scattered. Neither of my parents is here, since my dad had already flown out for my surgery, and my mom — well, 9/11 was three weeks ago, the nation is in a winter of fear, and I have all but ordered her to stay home.

How long will it be before I hear a human voice again — ten minutes? Thirty? Sixty? What will happen in between? I don't even know how to ask, so I am just floating along with the experience like a man riding a piece of driftwood down a river. When Cache hands me the headpiece I just look up at him, asking with my eyes whether I should put it on. My hands feel large and clumsy. I lift it up to my head where I think the implant is, and nothing happens. Where *is* it? I move it around and finally I feel it suction itself onto a spot above and behind my left ear, nearly an inch away from my best guess of where the implant was. How strange not to have known where it was! I let it go and it stays there, sticking to the side of my head. (See figure 4.)

Cache next hands me the processor, which is about the size of a pager. I fumble the end of the headpiece cord into a round slot on top of it. Becky removes its battery and plugs a serial cord into it from a laptop. I am now at the receiving end of a daisy chain of computers: laptop talks to processor, processor talks to implant, implant talks to me.

Talks? Or something like that.

As Becky watches over his shoulder, Cache taps a key on his keyboard. I suddenly hear a sharp, pure *beep* somewhere in my head. It's a single electrode being fired an inch and a half inside my skull. It surprises me so much that my head jerks back and my whole body seizes up. Out of the corner of my eye, I can see Margaret and

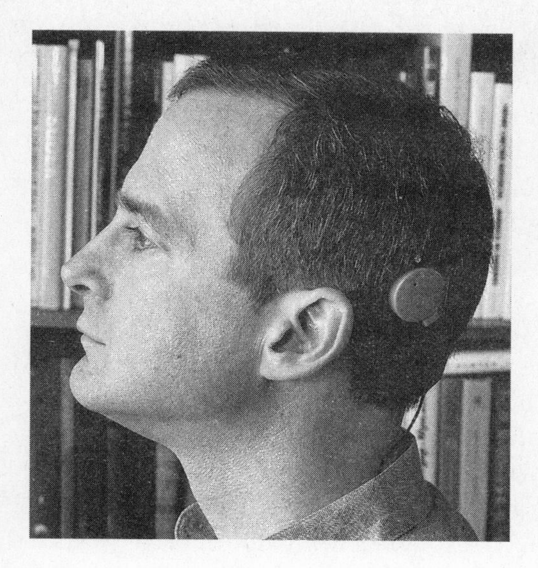

Figure 4. The headpiece. I had wondered whether it would glom on so hard it would mat my hair or abrade my skin, but in fact it sticks with pressure lighter than that of a single fingertip.

Paula laughing in joy and relief. They don't know what I've heard, but they can see I've heard *something.*

I haven't been activated yet, though. I'm just being calibrated. The next hour is a tedious series of beeps. This is mapping, a process designed to locate my comfort levels for stimulation in each electrode. Using his laptop as Becky looks on, Cache sends electrical current to various pairs of electrodes. Each time, I hear the current as a *beep* sound. Depending on where the pairs are in my cochlea, I hear *beeps* of various pitches. The higher the voltage, the louder the beep is to me. My job is to let Cache know when a given beep is getting too loud for comfort. With that information, Cache can set my maximum stimulation level — my *M-level* — for that electrode pair so that the computer never delivers more voltage to it than I find physically comfortable, regardless of how loud a given sound is.

Finally, Cache and Becky are satisfied. They play me the scale of all of my M-levels, eight *beeps* ascending from low to high. I watch on the screen as the computer shows when each electrode pair is being fired.

"The computer's playing my ear," I say, awed.

I am now an output device of the computer. In old DOS parlance, the user or programmer could direct a program's output to a particular external device by using cryptic little codes:

lpt1 Line Printer 1
tty Teletypewriter
com1 Communications Port 1

and so forth. Perhaps the programmers had to create a new output device:

hum Human

Then Cache turns and says to me, "The big moment."

He warns me that I may not like it. That it may sound robotic, or that voices may sound like Minnie Mouse. I nod. Deep down, I don't believe him. I think it'll sound better than that.

Then he hits his laptop's ENTER key.

Static. It's like when Murphy, the cyborg in *Robocop*, first opens his eyes. All he sees is TV snow. All I hear is static. Everything sounds awful: muddy and incomprehensible. There's a pervading roaring sound that I can't even begin to locate. I stammer out something just to hear my voice, and it sounds like rusty train wheels squeaking through mud.

I've got the expression of a man who's just swallowed what he thought was Pepsi only to find it's actually Pepto-Bismol. Cache and Becky do a few exercises to put my new ear through its paces. I close my eyes to eliminate lip-reading as they each recite the days of the week in turn. I can vaguely pick out the singsong cadence, but I can't be sure when one person has stopped and another has started. Even worse, I can't tell their voices apart.

Then we try assorted words. I get a few of them — "ice cream," "telephone" — but I'm wrong as often as right. "Give me a sentence," I say. I'd like to have something I can contextualize. I'm feeling like a man skidding down a hill, grabbing around for anything to slow the fall.

Cache says, "Zzzzzz szz szvizzz ur brfzzzzzz."

"Again," I say.

"Zzzzzz szz szvizzz ur brfzzzzzz."

I sigh. "A spinach and cheese omelet," I say. Everyone roars in delight — except me. I got it right, but I know that I'm doing it based on the cadence of the sentence and the one syllable I can actually feel that I have heard: the "br" in "breakfast." It's like solving a crossword puzzle. All I needed was one or two letters and a bit of context (it's midmorning, after all). I'm not actually *hearing* it.

"Now give me a sentence I can't predict," I say. Again I experience the woozling sensation that I have just learned corresponds to speech, but it's like squinting at a poster through yards of fog. "Again," I say. The words *color, is, black,* and *dog* surface somewhere in my mind, as if someone were telepathically beaming the words into my cortex. "Again," I say, trying for confirmation. Cache repeats the sentence a third time. I frown. "This can't be right, but what I think I'm hearing is, *What color is your black dog?*"

I open my eyes. Cache is smiling and nodding. "That's what I said."

It's hard for me to argue with this. The sentence defied my expectations, but I got it anyway. I *must* have heard it.

I scowl at him. "It doesn't feel like I heard you. It felt like guessing."

And it does. It feels like reading a page with half the letters whited out. One might be able to skate over it and get the gist, but it isn't going to feel like reading.

"It *will* get better," Becky says.

"It *will* get better," Cache says.

Margaret and Paula helpfully give me excited thumbs-up signs.

Better? *How?* I'm thinking: *Even if it gets twice as good as this, it's still going to be terrible.*

The session comes to a close. As I stand up, I'm so stiff that I have to crank my head back and forth a couple of times to unlock my neck. I pay the fee for being switched on and walk out on wobbly feet.

Numbly, I drive over to the office where I work. I don't want to go home. I want to go where people are, to check in, wander around trying out people's voices, and prove that I'm at least still alive in this new body I've found myself in.

The sound of the cars whipping past mine on El Camino Real upsets me badly. It isn't the deep, leathery rumble I'd heard all my life with hearing aids. Now it's a high-pitched *scree*, as if each car was squealing in pain.

I turn on the radio to its default station, National Public Radio. I haven't heard it in three months, and I've been longing to hear its announcers' lucid, flawless diction again. To hear National Public Radio is to be assured that there is a rational universe out there, with people who weigh both world events and their own thoughts with equal measure. But what I hear might as well be Esperanto. It sounds like a human voice, yet I cannot pick out a single word that I can recognize as English.

But the turn signal is okay. It's a firm, definite click, as familiar and reliable as castanets. I turn it on far ahead of each turn, just so I can hear *something* that sounds normal.

Before I go in the building, I steer myself in a wide circle around it so I can take a few deep breaths. There are large fibrous magnolia leaves scattered on the ground, turned brown and stiff. Absent-mindedly, I kick one.

It *tinkles.* As it skitters along the ground, it makes a tinny, tinfoily little noise as its edges scrape along the concrete. Disconsolate though I am, I find this deeply interesting. It brings out the six-year-old in me. As I make my way around the building, I go out of my way to kick leaves, sometimes booting a particularly noisy leaf ahead of me three or four times to get maximum entertainment value out of it. Each time, the leaf goes *clitter clitter clitter clitter.*

I go up to my office. As I clomp up the stairs I gasp a little in surprise at each footfall. I sound like a military troop invading the building.

The toilet flushing: an explosion. I back out of the stall at high speed, fumbling for the volume control at my waist with inexperienced fingers.

And then I talk to someone in my department. The leaves had sounded perfectly distinct, but I can't make any sense of his voice. After fifty thousand dollars' worth of work I can hear leaves, footsteps, and toilets, but not people.

And yet little sounds are weirdly clear. When I get home, I walk out to the backyard to check the tomatoes. As I step out the door, I'm brought up short. I'll be damned.

Crickets.

That rusty *cheep-cheep-cheep* sound, both so familiar and so strange.

For long minutes I stand there, framed in moonlight, listening.

The next morning is the beginning of my first full day in my bizarre new body. I get up and spend longer than I should getting dressed, hesitant to put on the processor. The headpiece is apparently happy to get to work: it sucks itself right into place. Finally, after spending way too long choosing my belt and shoes, I turn the processor on.

And there's a howling, high-pitched din all around me. I try to look in every possible direction simultaneously, attempting to place the source. I stare up at the smoke alarm and poke at it suspiciously with a broom handle. Then I interrogate the TV, the microwave, and the fridge. They all seem contented enough. But still: an enormous racket.

What the FUCK am I hearing? This can't be part of normal life. If I can't figure out what it is, I'm going to get upset.

I storm outside, hunting for clues. The noise just gets louder. My neighbor is rolling her bike out the door, heading for work. I bellow at her, "Is my smoke alarm going off?" Confused, she shakes her head. I look at Elvis on the front lawn: he's crouching under a bush. If it were the smoke alarm, his little ears would be flat against his head. They're not. This actually makes me *more* worried. Now I have *no* idea what is going on. I expand my search range, walk out to the street. To the right is a utility truck. To the left, on the other side of the street, is a man with . . . a leaf blower.

A leaf blower. It scared the crap out of me a hundred feet away, behind closed doors and windows.

There's no question that the implant delivers raw sound. I'm at *six* now, but it sounds more like *eleven*. It's like driving a V-8 with a loose steering wheel.

God, what a way to start the morning. If I could just close my eyes and listen to a little calm, measured NPR, I would feel better. But I know I can't, so I go to work. When I get there, I'm not feeling well. Dizzy. Pale. Cold sweat. It's clearly triggered by stimulation from the implant. I can't even begin to work. I put my head down on my desk and close my eyes. This sucks. I'm still deaf for all practical purposes, and now I'm dizzy again.

After a while I feel better, and bravely decide to go talk to Cheryl, our office administrator. I ask her about the timing of my upcoming move to an office down the hall. After listening to her voice for a minute or two, I blurt out the silliest thing imaginable: "You know, you sound . . . like a woman." And she does! Like Minnie Mouse, squeaky and staccato, but that's better than yesterday, when men sounded no different from women. Now I discover that the men I talk to sound, rather surprisingly, like themselves. All the women sound like Minnie Mouse. But I'm happy to have achieved gender differentiation. That's bound to be useful.

The day unfolds. I go upstairs to talk to a researcher about a literature search I'm helping him do at Stanford. I happily show him how the headpiece sticks to my head, and we get down to business. We talk. And it works out. He sounds rather odd, but I can understand him without having to hyperfocus. He uses proper names and I actually get them. It's the first reasonably relaxed, convivial conversation I've had in three months. I drag things out for an extra five minutes just to enjoy the sensation.

Toward the end of the day, in a fit of naive optimism, I try to call my mom on the phone. Reality strikes back. She sounds like a mournful wraith speaking in tongues. I can just barely make out a word here and there.

I say, "Mom, I just don't understand how I'm ever going to be able to make sense out of this."

She says, "A mmbf grrf better."

I hazard, "It might get better?"

She says, "It mmbf grrf better."

I say, "It may get better?"

She says, "It wlll grrf better."

I say, finally getting it, "It WILL get better."

But I haven't really heard her. I have extrapolated and guessed. I know the length of the sentence, I know the bisyllable at the end of it, and most of all, I know what my mom would say. In truth, I could have guessed it on the first try. But I demanded repeats, futilely attempting to have the experience of *hearing* it.

To celebrate my new ear, I go out to buy my first portable CD player. I want to play my familiar old CDs as a way of mapping my new auditory world onto my old one. Knowing how *Bolero* sounds — or, at any rate, *did* sound through hearing aids and cochleas missing most of their hair cells — will help me reconnect to reality, whatever exactly that is these days.

I start by going to Radio Shack to get a cable, which will enable me to connect the CD player directly to the processor. The processor has an audio input jack for just this purpose. I am greeted immediately by a young, attentive, and rather expressionless employee.

"What can I do for you?"

"I'd like to get a patch cable to connect to a CD player," I say.

"You're connecting it to a speaker?" he says.

I hesitate. How do I explain this? I decide to give him the short version, and let him ask questions to figure it out in his own way. I point to the processor's input jack at my waist. "I'm going to plug it into this."

But he doesn't ask any questions. He leads me to the back and rummages authoritatively among cables hanging in plastic bags. He hands me one consisting of three jacks on each end. I study it. "This doesn't look right. It should have only one plug on each end."

"You're going to plug it into a speaker?" he says again.

"Uh, no," I say. I point again to the processor at my waist, and then to the back of my head. "This is a bionic ear. The patch cable will go in here. Then the sound'll go into my head."

He simply nods and turns back to the cables on the wall. I'm a little befuddled. Maybe he has customers walking into the store all the time asking how to plug things into themselves. He picks out a cable and hands it to me.

"Can I try this out first?" I say. "I want to make sure it works."

He rustles up a CD player from the display case and slides a disc into it. I peek at the label. It's country and western. He keeps the player in his hands, which unnerves me because I don't know what the heck is going to happen. I entertain a brief vision of a searing pain in my head, followed by both me and my credit card dropping limply to the floor. Killed by George Strait.

Well, if I can't control the CD, at least I can yank the patch cable out really, really fast. I unobtrusively take hold of the end on my side just before he presses the PLAY button.

It's music! The sound quality isn't all that great, but the beat comes through clearly.

An hour later, I'm home with a patch cable and a new Walkman. As I sit down on the couch to listen, Elvis arches his back and rolls belly-up to greet me. It occurs to me that *there's no way he can hear the music.* If I were wearing headphones, he'd be able to hear whatever little bit of sound leaked out. But I'm plugged directly into the player. Its electrical output goes straight into the processor, which converts it to binary and passes it on to the implant. The implant decides which electrodes to trigger in my cochlea. There are no physical vibrations *anywhere.* All Elvis is ever going to hear is the hum of the player itself.

I'm hearing music that never actually exists as sound.

This could be evidence of a profound transformation in how human beings take in information from the world around them. Or it could just be a cozy domestic scene: a cyborg and his cat. *Bolero* zips by energetically, accelerating as it goes. Elvis emits a contented little cat sigh — I can feel his breath coming out of his nostrils — and lays his head on my arm.

A week or two after activation, the mad orchestra has dismissed most of its players. The implant masks the auditory hallucinations the way the sun blanks out the stars. When I take off the headpiece, I still hear the soft roar of a distant crowd. But no longer a jet engine, or a restaurant with a thousand patrons, or jazz drummers on speed.

It's as if my auditory cortex had been angrily saying to me, "If you won't give me sound, then I'm just going to make it up." Which it proceeded to do, endlessly, in inverse proportion to the loss. But now that it is being gorged with all it can take, it is happy again, and it has shut up.

The first night I realize that, I take off my clothes and go to sleep in a deep, blessed silence.

Two days later, I have my second mapping session. The first session is always just an approximation, a rough sketch, a setting of some basic parameters. Then they kick you out and give you a day or two to deal with the sheer shock of having a functional ear. The first-day map may be terrible, in fact it may bear very little resemblance to the map you will have a year later, but it's a start. Then they bring you back in to work on the map some more.

I want some objective information so I can compare my new ear to the old one, so I ask for a hearing test. I climb in the booth and Becky starts giving me tones. Some of the sounds are very faint indeed, but I know they're there, so I press the button that signals I've heard them. After just a few minutes, much earlier than usual, Becky throws open the door. In mock exasperation, she says, "Mike, where is your sensitivity dial?"

My sensitivity dial is one of the three dials on my processor — and it's the one I'm confused about. My hearing aids had had no equivalent to it. It controls the sensitivity of the microphone in the headpiece. I get that. What I don't get yet is how to use it in real life. When is high sensitivity good? When's it bad? Why do I even have control over that particular parameter? But just before this test I had turned it all the way up, figuring that more was better.

"It's set to max," I say. Then, seeing her demeanor, I add, "Is there a problem?"

"Yes and no," Becky says. "You're hearing sounds down to fifteen decibels."

Fifteen decibels. That is very, very faint — about the volume of a very soft whisper.

"We can increase your thresholds so you don't have to max your sensitivity," Becky says. She hauls me out of the booth and reattaches me to the computer for more mapping. More *beeps.* Then I'm back in the booth, and we go through the pure-tone testing again.

Then, without telling me how I've done on the pure tones, Becky starts a word recognition test. I am well familiar with it, having done it many times in my life. The words, as always, are as bland and white-bready as they can possibly be. It's an easy test.

"Hot dog," the testing booth says to me.

"Hot dog," I say.

cowboy

"Cowboy."

hot dog

"Hot dog."

airplane

"Airplane."

cowboy

"Cowboy."

hot dog

"Hot dog."

ice cream

"Ice cream."

At this point, I have the feeling I'm following Becky into fainter-sounding words than I've ever heard before. Theoretically, I shouldn't be able to tell this. Words will sound faint near a person's threshold, whatever their actual loudness is. But still — I know.

airplane

"Airplane."

cowboy

"Cowboy."

hot dog

I hesitate. "Bell bottom?"

ice cream

I cock my head. "I can hear it, but I'm not sure what it is."

After a few more words, the test ends. Cache invites me out of the booth. Becky shows me my new pure-tone audiogram, superimposed on top of my audiogram with hearing aids. An audiogram plots how loud sounds of various frequencies have to be before the patient can hear them. Sound loudness is measured in decibels, or dB. Roughly speaking, conversation is about 60 decibels. A rock concert is about 110 decibels. A person who can't hear sounds until they're up to about 40 dB is defined as having a moderate hearing loss.

My new audiogram, with a cochlear implant, is nearly a straight line going across all frequencies at the 25 dB level. It's the audiogram of a person with only a mild hearing loss.

"Is that good?" I say, knowing the answer but wanting to hear it anyway.

"Is it good?" Becky says. "Mike, it's *fantastic*."

My audiogram and my acuity for raw sound might be "fantastic," but in conversations amid the noise and confusion of real life, my hearing is bewilderingly poor. A few days after activation, I take a call from my bank about a discrepancy on my statement.

"Grmllar brum effiq anar," the phone says to me.

I frantically twist up the processor's volume dial. "Uh, could you say that again?"

"Grmllar brum effiq anar, rrrrm abrrr umurr burnum."

I pause to assess the situation. She might as well be speaking Tamil. Maybe she *is* speaking Tamil.

"I'm sorry, I'm hearing-impaired and I don't hear very well. Could you please slow down and say that again?"

"Grmllar . . . brum . . . effiq . . . ammar, arumm rerum orumm bvrrm."

My face starts to get warm.

"Look, I'm sorry, this just isn't working out. I'll try to handle this some other way."

"Umurr breemr corruar nrrrm, arrrum rrrrm effrm ommar trrm sssrm errumar prrrr, frrr arrr umurr etrrr ammar, orurrr tennar."

She clearly thinks that if she just says it in more detail, I will magically understand. I'm starting to feel like a little old lady being dragged across the street by a well-meaning Boy Scout.

"I know you're trying, but I'm sorry, I just can't hear you. Let me see if I can do this some other way."

"Ammmar grrrm trrrrm umurr errrm, brrm prrrm evarr emarr grum?"

I open my mouth, but can't think of anything to say.

"Umurr brrm errm ammar grrm enruum rrrrrm?"

Speechless, I hold the phone a foot away from my face and stare at it as if it's about to come to life and bite me. After a moment listening to it emit more babble, I hang up as softly as I can. Then I put my head down on my desk for a while. What's going to happen when the voice on the other end is a client?

Ten days post-activation. I visit my ex-girlfriend Ruth,* who is in town for the week on business. Ruth was my first real girlfriend when I was thirty, living in Austin, and still so clueless in bed that I would accidentally smack her head with my elbows while getting

* I've changed names to protect privacy, here and elsewhere.

up. Ruth is stout, cheerful, and mischievous, a *mensch*ette, a good human being all the way through.

We go to an Indian restaurant in Mountain View. I'm morose and irritable, because I'm not hearing very well. I'm terrified that I've reached the limits, that this is as good as it's going to get. Sure, I'm hearing raw sound, but in terms of comprehension, I'm still stumbling like a teenager trying to walk gracefully.

During the meal, I keep jumping.

BRRRANGLE

"What the heck is *that*?"

"It's the cash register behind you, Mike."

"Can't they make money more quietly?" I mutter.

CRRRASH

"What's *that*?"

"Somebody dropped glasses in the kitchen."

"The kitchen?" This is a novel idea to me: that hearing can reliably tell you about events that happen on the other side of walls. I have to probe this. "Do you *know* that's what it is, or are you just guessing?"

Ruth has to think this one over. It's a deep question in the epistemology of hearing.

"I'm pretty sure that's what it is."

Afterward we go back to her hotel. I've brought along my toothbrush. We know each other's bodies and desires, and we happen not to take either particularly seriously. It's just good for us to be together.

Except that today my body is different, and it confuses us both. For one thing, the processor has the effect of tying my shirt and pants together, since it is clipped both to the belt and to my undershirt. Kneeling before me, Ruth encounters the dilemma of where to begin disassembling me, and I'm almost as confused as she is. I pull up on the headpiece at the same time as she pulls down on the processor. The cord goes taut enough to vibrate under my shirt. I quickly let go of the headpiece and drop it down into my shirt.

Getting the processor off is easy after that, but then Ruth isn't sure whether to hand it back to me or put it on the floor, and I'm not sure either. If it's in my hand, how am I going to get my shirt off?

We finally settle for parking it on the floor. Clothes go fluttering in various directions: we know how to do *this,* at any rate. Finally I haul up the processor and attach the headpiece. Holding the processor in one hand, and Ruth's hand in the other hand, I lead the way to bed.

As we bounce into bed on our hands and knees, a perplexing question occurs to me. The processor is designed to be held in place by a belt.

I'm not wearing a belt. Or anything.

So *where does it go?*

Can I balance it on my back? Not too promising; it's going to get knocked off pretty fast. What about on the headboard of the bed? No luck; the bed doesn't have a headboard big enough to offer a ledge. Next to us, on the bed? Not so good, either; there's no way to hold the headpiece in place.

Well, two forces are going to compete here, desire and magnetism, and may the better fundamental force win. By this time I'm past caring. I park the processor on the bed sheet, to my left. It'll just have to fend for itself if we roll on top of it. Presumably someone considered this possibility when engineering the aluminum case.

SAS, the software I'm using at the moment, has no particular problem translating my auditory experience after this point, which goes something like this:

errr!
mmmph!
oof!
=smooch=
ugggh ugggh ugggh ugggh —
blip *vroooo*
(silence)

After a while, I fumble around the pillow for the headpiece and reattach it. For the rest of the evening, it will continue to fall off and be put back on. There are two magnets in the system, one in the headpiece, one in me, and they are so well calibrated to each other that the headpiece clings to my head with only the softest pressure — less than the gentle touch of a finger. That's good, because it keeps my skin from getting sore, but it's also bad, because the slightest tug will pull it off.

"Tell me about what's going on in Austin," I murmur, addressing some smooth part of Ruth's side.

"Arahjst brok ip whaguy isseeeng in Austin."

"Uh, try that again?"

"ARAHJST BROK IP WHAGUY ISSEEENG IN AUSTIN."

"Volume doesn't help," I say. "Remember, I can hear sounds softer than I could before." Then I hit on a brilliant idea. "Ruth, talk softly."

"I just broke up with the guy I was seeing in Austin."

I say, "You just broke up with the guy you were seeing in Austin."

"He was a lot of fun, but in the end I just had to tell'm arake ewalk."

"You just had to tell him . . ." I prompt.

"To take a walk."

And that's the way it goes from then on. It's not perfect, but we manage to have an intelligible conversation, the two of us in the dark, the little green light on my processor occasionally flashing companionably along with us.

We find that the green light is too good not to play with. When I crank the sensitivity up, it flashes in synchrony with any sound it hears. I hold the processor up in the dark. "Hello," I say.

blink blink

Ruth laughs, and the processor blinks back in a complicated little storm of varying intensities of green.

"Fourscore and seven years ago," I say, triggering off another round of blinking. We both laugh. It's infectious: when *we* laugh, *it* laughs.

Then I pull the headpiece off. Immediately, the green light becomes a forlornly blinking red light.

Awww, it misses me.

Then a thought occurs to me. "Hey, Ruth," I say, half jokingly. "Want to see the scar?"

"Sure," she says.

I roll on my right side and scoot backwards in her direction. I angle my head down, almost as if preparing to meditate, and submit quietly as her fingers probe my hair above and behind my ear. She finds the implant and touches it gently, running her fingers along its slightly raised outline. I sigh deeply and go very still. This is what I want: for a woman to gently touch this part of my body where I have so recently been torn open and then reassembled into something I still barely recognize. This part of me still feels alien, other, not-me. Her touch is a kind of psychic suturing, helping me along in the process of integrating it into myself. My body is everything she feels, scar and metal and flesh, all together.

5. Forget About Reality

> . . . The commands you type into a computer are a kind of speech that doesn't so much communicate as *make things happen,* directly and ineluctably, the same way pulling a trigger does. They are incantations, in other words . . . the logic of the incantation is rapidly permeating the fabric of our lives.
>
> —JULIAN DIBBELL, *My Tiny Life*

> Your tale, sir, would cure deafness.
>
> — SHAKESPEARE, *The Tempest*

IN A DREAM I stumbled in a field, and fell. When I revisit that field in my mind's eye, I can see that it consists of fibers arranged in orderly rows. It is the field of cell-sized hairs in my cochlea (see figure 5). I can look down upon it to see three rows of V-shaped outer hair cells and one row of I-shaped inner hair cells.

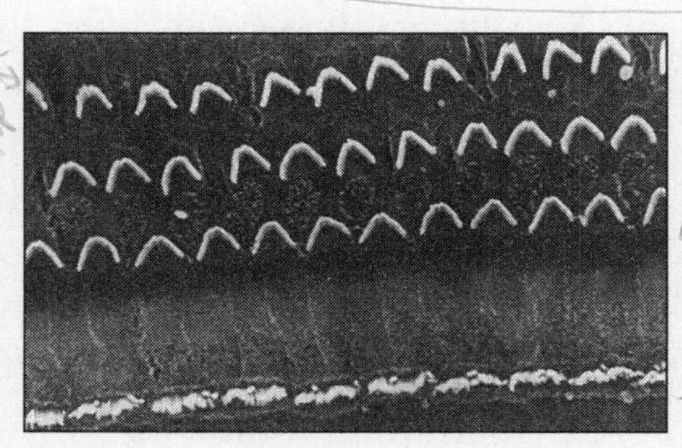

Figure 5

The field is tiny: each hair cell is eight or nine thousandths of a millimeter wide. By comparison, a human hair is 80–100 thousandths of a millimeter wide.

I descend to the field and walk up to one of the *V*'s, which comes up to my chest. I am ten-thousandths of a millimeter tall, standing on top of one of my outer hair cells. The fibers growing out of it are *stereocilia,* made of protein, leaning together in a cluster as elegant and brittle as blown glass (figure 6).

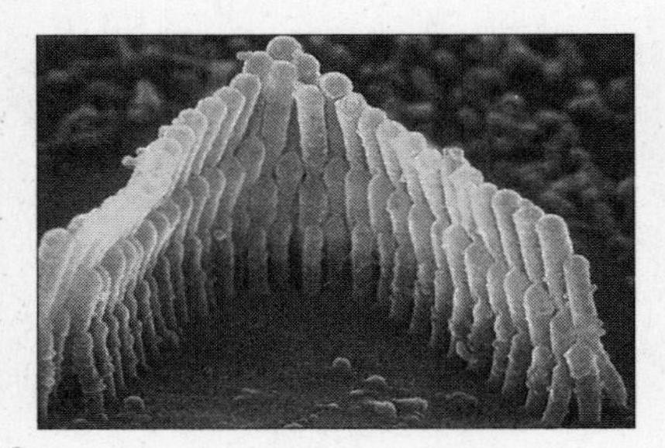

Figure 6. A close-up picture of the top of an outer hair cell. The fibers, called *stereocilia,* flex in response to sound waves.

This is Eden, a garden of harmony. The hair cells sit atop the *basilar membrane,* which runs the length of the cochlea. The basilar membrane undulates below my feet, elastic, oceanic. The wave motion comes from the eardrum and the three tiny bones connecting it to the cochlea, kilometers away on my scale. All around me the stereocilia sway back and forth like kelp on a sea floor. Flashes of electricity glow and fade beneath my feet.

To my right and left stretch 12,500 of the outer hair cells and 3,500 of the inner hair cells, disappearing in each direction around the bend of the great spiral going from base to apex. The inner hair cells pick up the wave motion, muster up floods of neurotransmitters, and send streams of electricity to my brain. The outer hair cells receive signals *from* the brain that cause them to stiffen and relax. If a very faint sound comes in, triggering just a few of the inner hair cells, the brain tells the outer hair cells to stiffen in such a way as to cause *more* inner hair cells to fire, boosting the system's sensitivity. They can interact because a tight membrane is draped over them both (it has been peeled off in the photos). When the outer hair cells stiffen, the membrane tugs on the inner hair cells, making more of them fire. The ear is not a passive organ. It responds actively to the world to shape sensation more to its liking, the hair cells harmonizing in a complex and lovely interactive dance.

But then the scene shifts and changes. Figure 7 shows what my stereocilia actually look like.

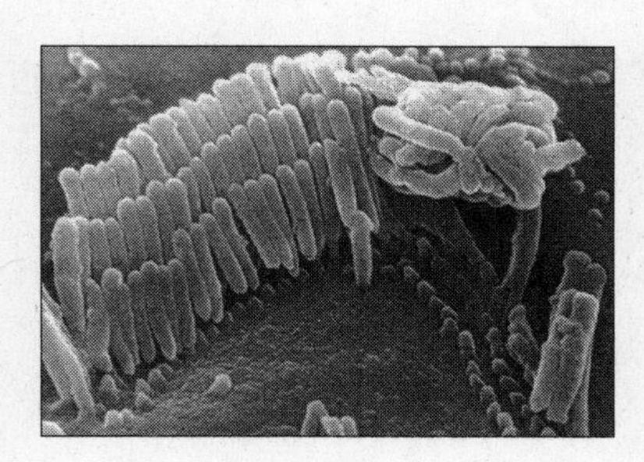

Figure 7. A badly damaged outer hair cell.

Eden is destroyed. The rubella virus stunted my ear's stereocilia, blew them apart, tore them loose from the cell surfaces. No more electrical impulses; my cochlea is dark and silent.

This is the inner ear I made do with for thirty-six years, with hearing aids pumping in sound at such high volumes that the few remaining intact clusters were made to move by sheer sonic force. And then on July 7, 2001, those clusters collapsed as well. The reason: unknown. All I know is that my ear died, and I fell.

And then the computer penetrated my body. In my vision I see a vast cable, kilometers long and the diameter of the Alaskan pipeline on my scale, being snaked through the lower chamber of my cochlea. Sixteen electrodes lie along its length, pointing toward the center of the cochlea, the *modiolus,* where the nerves are bundled together in trunk lines. The electrodes don't point toward the hair cells, which are irrelevant now. Dead keys on a piano. Bypass them. Instead, the electrodes trigger the nerve endings in the modiolus.

But the sequence in which the electrodes are fired is all-important. Seat an idiot at a piano and all you get is cacophony. For euphony you need to understand the neural code: the way the body triggers the nerve endings in life. The cochlea has three mechanisms for converting sound into nerve impulses, called *rate coding*, *place coding*, and *phase coding*. Place coding happens to be the easiest to replicate with a string of implanted electrodes, because from a place coding perspective, the cochlea resembles a piano keyboard in a spiral. Hair cells at the base of the cochlea resonate to high frequencies; ones at the apex, to low frequencies. The electrode array can therefore simulate the place coding mechanism by firing electrodes in the appropriate places. High frequencies are transmitted by firing electrodes at the base of the cochlea; low frequencies, by firing electrodes at the apex. The other two mechanisms, rate coding and phase coding, are so much more difficult to replicate electrically that the engineers have focused on place coding. But is replicating only one of the ear's mechanisms enough to do the job? The brain is so flexible — so eager to deal with whatever information it gets — that the answer, more or less, is yes. So the electrode array plays the cochlea like a piano.

That is, a very small and very complex piano. Most sounds consist of a jumble of frequencies. A normal cochlea uses physical mechanisms to separate out the frequencies the way a coin sorter rattles coins into piles. A cochlear implant, however, has to do the task with binary logic, digitally taking sound apart and figuring out which electrodes to fire on the array in every passing millisecond. The software that manages this process is one of *the* monumental achievements of bionics. Here is a very small piece of it, written in a language called C.

```
DualLoopAGC() {
    int incr;
    if (Env > CslowInt) {
        /* attack mode */
        int FastThresh = qMultClip(CslowInt,dBplus8,3);
        int EnvLimit;
        if (Env > FastThresh) {
            incr = 0;
```

```
} else {
      /* incr = 3; */
      incr = 2; /* 3-8-2000 based on input from
            Jason Lee and Michael Stone */
      FastRecovery();
}
```

This particular bit of code is part of the *automatic gain control* subroutine. In a deaf ear there are no physical mechanisms to amplify soft sounds and damp loud ones, so the software fiddles with its own output to achieve the same end. This is more than just a bit of fine-tuning. A rock concert is not just ten or twenty times louder than ordinary conversation; it is *hundreds of thousands* of times louder. If the amount of electricity being pumped into me increased proportionately, it would, at the very least, melt the electrode array and fry my cochlea. So the code vigilantly monitors how loud the world is, and ensures that the voltage always grows more slowly than the volume. This kind of logic is what makes me a *cybernetic organism,* an organic creature whose body is controlled by algorithmic rules.

(When I first read this code, I was eerily aware that these very instructions were being executed *right now,* over and over, thousands of times per second, in my processor and inside my head. They were what enabled me to hear the paper rustling as I paged through it, my own voice muttering lines here and there. I was reading my own software.)

Since only one of the three neural mechanisms is being reproduced, the software's version of reality is by definition impoverished, monochrome, coloring-book simple. Or rather, *both* versions of the software are. At activation I was given two computer programs, called SAS and CIS, to choose from in controlling the electrode array. I could switch back and forth between them by thumbing a dial on my processor. While they both played my cochlea like a piano, they had completely different ways of hitting the "keys." SAS, or *S*imultaneous *A*nalog *S*timulation, fed current to all of the electrodes all the time, giving me continuous stimulation along the entire length of the electrode array. And it was *analog* stimulation, meaning that the current levels at each electrode were smoothly increased or decreased rather than switched on and off.

On the other hand, CIS, *C*ontinuous *I*nterleaved *S*ampling, was digital. At any given instant, only one electrode was being fired. CIS shuttled rapidly among the electrodes, firing them at a rate of 833 per second, giving me the illusion of continuous stimulation. It worked on the same principle as television, where the electron gun sweeps so rapidly across the screen that the eye perceives continuous motion.

Why even bother to give me two completely different ways of controlling the electrode array? Why not just decide which is better, and give me that one? But they had been developed by different teams with different ideas, and studies had shown that users broke more or less evenly when given a choice between them. There was perplexity in the halls of science over how best to represent sound, so I was invited to experiment. It was like handing a musical illiterate a guitar and two manuals with different philosophies of how to play it, and saying, "Here. *You* decide."

So over the next few weeks, I experimented. I thumbed my dials endlessly. Windchimes on CIS. Windchimes on SAS. Mom's voice on CIS. Mom's voice on SAS. *Me* on CIS. Me on SAS. I soon discovered that CIS and SAS had very different ways indeed of handing me the world. CIS, the first program I had used at activation, gave me *Zzzzzz szz szvizzz ur brfzzzzzz.* SAS gave me *BLUH DHYOU AV R BRKFSSS.* CIS made the world sound quiet, metallic, and tinny. SAS made it sound big, blocky, and fuzzy. CIS minced. SAS galumphed. CIS fed me sound daintily, with chopsticks. SAS threw it at me in brawny shovelfuls.

One new version of the world would be unsettling enough. If the sky is suddenly always green, you can at least decide to accept that as reality and do your best to get used to it. But if you have a choice between worlds where the sky is green in one and pink in the other, your sense of reality goes right out the window. I had never heard the world mincing *or* galumphing, chopsticked *or* shoveled. To be sure, the implant delivered raw decibels. I could hear clocks ticking across a room. But I did not *feel* like a hearing person. A hearing person? Hah! I was the receptor of a flood of data, which I was constantly stitching into meaningful language a half-second or so after I actually heard it. And my performance outside the testing booth was terrible. With even minor background noise, or on the phone, I lost people's words like sawdust in the wind. All I knew was that I had two versions of reality, and they both sounded wrong.

A few days after activation, I discovered on CIS that the pages of a report I was editing were making very interesting sounds as I turned them. I got a crisp little rustle each time, which was what I expected, but there was also a tinkling *binggg* sound coming on its heels like an echo, which I most definitely didn't expect.

Experiment time. I gathered up the whole report, about fifty pages, and dropped it on the desk.

blap-BINGGG

In my experience paper made sounds like *blap*, *snip*, and *vrrrrr*, and if rudely treated, *szzzzz*. It didn't go *bingggg*.

Well, *this* paper did. I rattled three or four pages:

szzzz-bing szzzz-bing szzzz-bing

It was like shaking the paper and seeing a rainbow halo emerge unsteadily from around its edges.

So that was what paper sounded like on CIS. I switched to SAS and rustled the paper some more. No *binggg* this time.

Did that mean SAS was "better"? More "right"? *I didn't know.* Perhaps CIS was giving me additional auditory information that I hadn't learned to process yet. The electrode array was stimulating areas of my cochlea that had never had hair cells. Maybe some component of the paper's rustling was sounding like *binggg* to me because my auditory cortex didn't know how else to interpret it.

Or maybe not. Maybe it was just a weirdness of CIS, and SAS was giving me a more authentic auditory representation.

Or maybe rattled paper really did go *binggg* and I was only now discovering it, at age thirty-six.

In effect, I was taking a lab course in the philosophy of radical skepticism. In 1740 David Hume had argued that the senses give us only interpretations of reality, leaving us — in the end — completely ignorant of what reality actually is. He had dismissed the argument that people generally agree on what reality is. Consensus is not proof, he'd said. It's just consensus. All we can know for certain is what our senses *think* reality is.

David Hume would have loved the idea of cochlear implants: sense organs that can be told to think anything. But Hume didn't have to live his theories — he could just sit in his study in Scotland and write. Two hundred and sixty-one years later, *I* was living his theories. All I knew "for certain" was how two completely different kinds of software interpreted the world. It was driving me crazy.

CIS and SAS were driving me crazy because while growing up, I had so much wanted to hear the world the way it *really was.* I had been incredibly fussy about finding the *right* hearing aid. When I was in my teens I tried a hearing aid made by a company named Widex and had loved it immediately. The Widex gave sound the kind of punch and character I wanted. I wore it long after it went out of date, because all of the newfangled digital hearing aids hitting the market in the 1980s sounded wrong — too subdued, too quiet, too hollow. The digital aids had *ideas* about reality. They had a mania for things like *peak clipping,* which consisted of computationally smoothing out the sound to make it more even. On the other hand, the Widex was just an amplifier that gave me the world straight and true.

Of course, as Hume would have immediately pointed out if he'd ever taken a course in electrical engineering, the Widex's output was also an interpretation of reality. With every specification of *this* microphone and not *that, this* tubing and not *that, this* resistor and not *that,* its engineers had built a cumulative set of choices about reality into its design. The result was a hearing aid that overamplified certain frequencies as an inherent property of its hardware, a common problem in aids of that era. But by great good luck, the Widex's frequency peaks just happened to coincide with the frequencies that I heard particularly well. The firestorm of the rubella had left random areas of my cochlea relatively unharmed. The Widex's design weaknesses fit into my auditory strengths, yin into yang, male plug into female socket, and the first time I put it on I felt a great burst of rightness, akin to the joy a tennis player feels when the ball hits the racquet in exactly the right place. The Widex hit the sweet spot of my ear. At that moment, my beliefs about the auditory world became set in glass.

It was strange that I should be so stubborn about perceiving the world in one and only one way, because the exact thing I loved about computers was their infinite malleability, their ability to create worlds out of imagination. In *My Tiny Life,* Julian Dibbell argues that computer programmers are akin to magicians because they write words that actually make things happen. *Let X=1,* a programmer can say, and behold, X *is* 1. *Let there be light,* and behold, there is light. Or darkness: say *DEL *.** in the proper context and you can wipe out all of the information on your hard disk. When Prospero, the magician in Shakespeare's *The Tempest,* becomes annoyed when his daughter's attention wanders, she placates him by saying, "Your tale, sir, would cure deafness." What an extraordinary idea: to tell a story where the words *themselves* have such power that they can bring the ruined ear back to life. This is what Dibbell means by the phrase "the logic of the incantation." As a magician, Prospero has such a power. He can cast spells, which are words that act on the world to make things happen.

So can programmers. It is actually possible, with computers, to have powers once existing only in myth and legend. SAS and CIS were computer programs, incantations, logical sequences of commands that the computer faithfully recited and executed line by line. They did not cure my deafness, for they could not make my hair cells regrow, but nonetheless they made me hear.

As a programmer, I found this unnerving. All my life, the magic of the computer had stayed inside the computer. My body was still my own. Augmented, to be sure, but still my own. Strand me on a desert island and I could still hear, at least a little bit, even without hearing aids. But now, in my desert-island fantasies I was mournfully clutching one end of a very, very long extension cord. I needed the electricity that made the incantations of CIS and SAS recite themselves over and over again, calling my auditory world into existence by a sustained act of verbal will. The hardware of the implant was necessary, but it was not the essence of my hearing, any more than ink and paper are the essence of a book. The essence of the implant was *language*, and the proof was that different incantations put me in different worlds. I was quite literally spellbound by the logic of the incantation.

But it was not so obvious how the spells should be cast. The parameters of each program could be adjusted endlessly. M-levels. T-levels. Dynamic range. Number of electrodes in use. Volume. Sensitivity. All together, I had not two but approximately 230,000 versions of reality to choose from.* During my first two mapping sessions Becky and I had had time to try only eight or ten of them. The process seemed so haphazard. "Let's try this." "Let's try that." What were the odds that we could find my ideal settings, the one *right* version of the world that I had heard long ago through primitive electronics? Nearly zero, it seemed. That world had disappeared forever. No more hair cells; no more sweet spots to hit. And code that could do anything with my nerve endings that it wanted.

The day I went deaf, I also became dizzy. The cochlea controls balance as well as hearing, a fact that becomes less surprising when one recalls that hair cells are exquisitely sensitive to motion. The cochlea has three loops attached to its upper end, each oriented in a different plane. They too are filled with hair cells. The slightest motion of the head or body causes the hair cells to move, and orientation signals flood through nerve pathways to the brain.

Not only had I lost the feeling that the auditory world enveloped me, but I had also lost the feeling that the physical world was fixed

* The number is actually much higher, but in my calculations I excluded extreme settings such as maximum volume or zero dynamic range.

and stable. I had no trouble walking or driving, but I felt slightly drunk much of the time. It's common to feel dizzy upon activation, but not common to feel dizzy for weeks afterward. Since the balance problem had started before the surgery, that ruled out the surgery itself as a cause. My cochlea hadn't seemed to mind having a foreign body stuffed inside it. Activation, though, had started up the wooziness again. My cochlea was clearly unhappy about being electrified.

That was unsettling enough, but whenever I felt especially unbalanced — the sensation came and went — the world sounded even more vague and fuzzy than usual, and no amount of fussing with my controls would help. Not only was my balance system fluctuating, so was my *hearing*. But how could that be possible? The computer was supposed to override the vagaries of my flesh by directly controlling my nerve endings. My hearing *couldn't* fluctuate, yet it was. Living in this body was like an endless waking dream where the world shifted and changed without warning. It was oddly reminiscent of my childhood.

I put the question to Dr. Roberson and he raised his hands in bafflement. There was simply no explanation for it. Apparently I still lived in a human body that had its own stubborn ways of doing things. My computer and my body would just have to figure out how to get along.

Somehow, I had to take the bizarrely changed flow of information from my senses and construct a world I could live with. But how to do that? There was one possible path, which I'd discovered years ago in the most surprising way imaginable. When I was a graduate student in the late 1990s, I'd been depressed enough to sign myself up for group therapy. Suffice it to say that graduate school sucks, and I needed help dealing with that fact. I couldn't hear well enough to understand the people on the other side of the circle, so I'd brought in an FM system, which consisted of a small radio transmitter and a small radio receiver that I could hook up to my hearing aids. Wherever the transmitter was, so were my ears.

This meant that before anyone could speak, they had to have the transmitter passed around the circle to them. I shudder now to think how badly it cramped the group's dynamics. They no doubt felt the passive ill will that comes of having to carry the wounded: a diffuse, untargetable resentment. My unease over the matter made me defensive, spiky, brittle. But I heard. And I listened.

And then one day the transmitter's batteries died. I packed it away and resigned myself to a wasted session. But, to my astonishment, I *could* hear the people on the other side of the circle. It was even more surprising because when the batteries had died before, I couldn't hear them. Something important had changed. But what?

What had changed, I suddenly realized, was my ability to listen. Not to hear, but to *listen.* When I joined the group I had believed that I suffered more from my little miseries than other people did. I would think, when someone else was talking, "You're saying the same things as I am, but I feel worse about them than you do." A kind of vanity. But as time went on I slowly came to understand that I was not unique. I saw them mumble shamefacedly about never getting laid, I saw them mourn breakups, I saw them cry. I began to realize, *Oh. I am like them.* And that enabled me to *be* there, to feel with and for them, instead of mentally twiddling my thumbs in my little castle that only the loudest sounds could penetrate. It was only when the FM technology failed that I realized that I had opened a lot of that castle's windows. I was able to hear astonishingly better because of it. I still remember that great burst of illumination, that breakthrough: I could upgrade my mental *software!* I could hear better by becoming a better *person!*

After that I'd used the FM system much less. It was then that my technology fetish had begun to fade. The gratification of upgrading my technology diminished. Upgrading *myself* was hard, slow, subtle work, but it had the enduring satisfaction of true craft.

And so, in the fall of 2001, I realized what I would have to do. I would have to complete the process I had started in group therapy. I would have to become emotionally open to what I heard, instead of fighting against it. If I didn't, I would reach only a fraction of my potential, both auditory and emotional. I needed every last decibel for getting back into Eden. Steroids had shown me the way by briefly making me into a person who did not hide and could not lie, but I could not take them again. I would have to get back to that place on my own.

I had hoped to hear the world whole and full — a door opening to reveal a blinding light — but now I was grudgingly realizing that my world would still be fragmentary and partial. Very well: *forget about reality.* Hearing with a cochlear implant, I realized in the third or fourth week post-activation, was going to be like a stone skipping across the surface of a lake. I would have to learn to glide over the soundstream, not always fully in contact with it but getting the general meaning. I would have to learn to backfill the incomplete information in my mind. I would have to give up the expectation that it would truly feel like hearing, and learn to use the implant as a tool that would enable me to do something which resembled hearing. It would not *be* hearing. It would just be *equivalent* to hearing.

How bizarre.

6. The Computer Reprograms Me

> Now all he needed was to find some human emotion in the tangle of plastic, wire and atomic metal that was fused to the remains of his flesh . . .
>
> — Wonderfully melodramatic back cover copy of Martin Caidin's *Cyborg*

FALL 2001. The air grew damper and cooler as the days waned and Halloween approached. The first few days of fall have always made me feel like a stranger to myself. I have a summer *self* and a winter *self,* and each time the world moves from one season to the other I feel an internal shift resetting the variables of my consciousness to different values. And then I feel like myself again. But it is always eerily strange that I have to change in order to stay the same.

This year, the process of reacquiring my winter self was a small wheel rolling around within a larger wheel. When would I forget the computer buzzing away in my head, experiencing it as a part of my body as normal as my heart or my liver? I was Mike *plus* something new and strange. I was constantly aware of the headpiece magnetically clinging to my skull. The faint tickle of the cord on my neck, the way it pulled gently when I craned my head one way or another, briefly pulling the magnet a millimeter or two off center. The way I could lift it half a centimeter or so off my head without losing the signal. The fact that my ears were now run by a control panel at my waist.

In *Cyborg,* Rudy Wells had guided Steve Austin through learning how his new body worked. In my own life, that task was divided among three people. There was my mom, who knew cochlear implants well because she had worked at Summit Speech School for decades; there was Becky, my audiologist; and there was Mike Faltys, the chief engineer at Advanced Bionics, whom I met on my first trip there some months later. On our first encounter, during a staff meeting, Mike Faltys had taken me through a high-speed Powerpoint presentation on the implant electronics. It had gone way over my head, bristling with diagrams and technical terms, and I'd inwardly prayed that I wouldn't need to communicate with *this* guy. But on my next visit we'd talked in his office, and he had seemed touched that I'd written about the blinking light on the processor. "I know exactly why that light blinks," he'd said, blinking a little himself, and the conversation branched and grew until we were talking about poetry and music, then William Blake and the doors of perception, and finally about whether one human being can ever truly know the experience of another. I sensed a certain wistfulness about him underneath that avalanche of technical terms, a feeling of being an alien in a world of humans, shy and eccentric yet adroit, driven to create machines that were beautiful yet still grounded in the realities of blood and bone and spirit. Mike turned out to be a superb explainer, and soon we were laughing and joking around.

From Mike I learned that my hearing had not been *restored,* it had been *replaced* with an entirely new system that had entirely new rules. One mechanism instead of three. A choice between analog and digital stimulation. And the underlying hardware was profoundly different from my original specifications. The radio signal going through my skin from the headpiece to the implant carried 1,113,636 bits per second of data. That amounted to one megabyte every 7.5 seconds, or enough to fill up a floppy disk in about 11 seconds. If things were very quiet, most of those bits would be zeros. If things were noisy, the bits would be a complicated pattern of zeros and ones. In other words:

ELVIS: *Meow.*
PROCESSOR: 10010100110000010100101011110010100101100110111.
ME: Aw, kitty, are you hungry?

The job of the chips inside the implant was to take all those 1s and 0s and decide which electrodes on the array to fire. I had assumed that those chips would be very "dumb," on the theory that engineers would locate the bulk of the computational power outside the body, in the processor, where it could be easily upgraded. The big computer would just tell the little computer what to do. That was true to a large extent, Mike explained to me, but there *were* in fact real smarts in the implant. The physics of radio waves imposed limits on how much data could be sent through the skin. To overcome that, he and his fellow engineers had made the implant just smart enough so that it could accept the broad "outlines" of sound from the processor and calculate some of the missing details on its own.

So a fair amount of computational work was going on inside my head as well as outside. The two chips in the implant together had about 140,000 transistors, making the implant approximately comparable to Intel's 286 microprocessor, which had 134,000 transistors when it was released in 1982. (Computers with Intel 286 microprocessors were the last ones that most computer manufacturers sold without the Windows operating system.) I now had roughly as much processing power in my head as in the desktop computer I'd had when I started graduate school.*

* *Very* roughly. I am exercising considerable license here. Like today's Pentiums, Intel's 286 was a general-purpose microprocessor designed to handle a wide variety of tasks. On the other hand, the chips in the implant are custom-designed to carry out only a few tasks, but to do them fast and efficiently. It's like comparing a jackknife stuffed with accessories (e.g., a 286) to a scalpel (e.g., the chips in my head). The scalpel does only one thing, but it does that one thing extremely well. Unlike a 286, the chips in my head could not run an operating system, recompute a spreadsheet, or do word processing (my post-op joke notwithstanding). On the other hand, because they are specialized, they can handle the computational load of controlling the electrode array faster than a 286 could.

The technological achievement was dazzling. But it didn't match a normal ear. Of the 15,000 hair cells in a healthy cochlea, about 3,500 of them — the I-shaped inner hair cells — directly transfer information to the brain. (The outer hair cells, as explained previously, support the work of the inner hair cells.) My cochlear implant had replaced those 3,500 hair cells with 16 electrode contacts. That was a reduction factor of *220 to 1.*

I didn't know about that reduction factor yet, in the fall of 2001. All I knew was that I heard static and mush. I had most definitely not reacquired my *self.* I felt incomplete, unfinished, a half-built cyborg with wires and springs sticking out. The radio and phone were still so hard to understand that neither of them had become a natural part of my life. Most people sounded like the teacher Miss Othmar in the *Peanuts* cartoon specials: muddy, orotund, unclear. I saw lips move, I heard sounds, but they didn't translate into words I could understand. It was wearyingly frustrating to have to ask people to repeat half of what they said, and still not get it half the time. Often I had to fall back on the desperate expedient of pretending to have understood. This was something I'd learned to avoid, because a lifetime of living with hearing loss had taught me that people weren't fooled by it. But I was just too besieged and embarrassed to try to chase down every single sentence. I had to ration my energy for the ones I thought were important.

The day of my one-month mapping, I was pissed. The world seemed drab, narrow, and confining. My ears didn't sound very good; my job was not particularly exciting; a woman whom I was interested in had just written, at the last minute, to postpone our date by a week. For the three months I was deaf, the normal rules of engagement with life had been suspended. But now I was hearing again. *Not* well. Back to being alone. Back to the same old struggle to hear and be heard.

I was finally beginning to understand the anger Steve Austin went through as he slowly adapted to his new arms and legs. "The arm is coming along fine, isn't it?" Steve had demanded of Rudy

Wells. "Then what the hell's the matter with the legs? Why can't they work out that feedback problem?" And then he had sent everything on the table crashing to the floor.

I was angry because I was afraid. Afraid that a new map wouldn't improve matters and that I'd have to spend the rest of my life in a blurred auditory universe.

"Pissed, pissed, pissed, pissed, pissed, pissed," I muttered to myself as I drove to the California Ear Institute. Working myself up into a fine little rage.

Half the fun of swearing is hearing it. The word *fuck* is satisfying because it is verbal dynamite. *Piss* is sibilant and intense. But I couldn't get even these little satisfactions. On SAS, *fuck* translated as a lame *fuh; piss* had all the impact of a deflating tire. CIS was even worse. It made me sound like a dyspeptic mouse.

Which just pissed me off even more. In the waiting room, I visualized myself throwing the processor out the window into the parking lot. It was just the right size for a satisfying windup and hurl.

I greeted Becky with a glare. I unloaded: my hearing sucks, I feel like I'm losing all the high frequencies, everything sounds mumbly and vague, there's no crispness, let alone clarity. Unruffled, Becky serenely plugged me into the computer and we began the tedious process of remapping. It was exactly like an eye test. Which is louder, Sound 1 or Sound 2? Sound 1, I said. Well, no, maybe it's Sound 2. Give them to me again.

This went on for a long time. Then Becky fussed with the computer and presented me with a new map, the result of all the sound-by-sound comparisons we'd done. I'd been clever: I had brought a tape player and two books on tape, *Piglet Is Entirely Surrounded by Water* and *Stuart Little.* With their known and exactly repeatable voices, they were baselines against which I could compare new maps.

I listened carefully to *Piglet.* "It sounds a little less bass," I said. "But still very mumbly."

We tried four or five variations on the map, but without much improvement. "I know my audiogram *says* I'm getting the high pitches," I said. "But I don't feel like I'm hearing them. It's like something's washing them out."

"Let's try turning off some of the electrodes," Becky said. "You're doing well on SAS, but maybe you're getting interactions between some of the electrodes."

So she tried turning off one electrode at a time. Over and over again, I listened to my tapes, assessing the clarity of the voices. Bit by bit, things got clearer. Things seemed to sound best when electrodes near the tip of the electrode array were turned off, so we focused on that area, trying out various combinations of switched-off electrodes.

It was when Becky turned off a pair of electrodes second from the tip of the array that I said, "All right, that sounds better."

And it did. Now everything sounded robotic and artificial — and that was an improvement over the aural sludge I had before. Now it sounded more like I was getting a clear signal I could do something with.

On the way home, I played with phonemes, especially fricatives and sibilants. The word *pissed* had just the right combination of sounds I wanted.

"Pissed, pissed, pissed, pissed, pissed, pissed," I sang to myself happily. Finally hearing the *S* as an *S*, and the *D* as a *D*.

By now I found myself gravitating to SAS. CIS had an annoying, burbling, bell-like quality. It sounded thin and tinny, and it was a pest, constantly presenting me with tinkling *binggg* sounds that had no apparent provenance in reality. On the other hand, SAS had a straightforward, bold, and blocky sound, an algorithm that gave me the world without game-playing. CIS seemed just too damn *coy*. But most of all, the world sounded somewhat more *right* with SAS. My own voice sounded deeper and fuller on SAS, whereas CIS made me feel embarrassingly alto. Note to software designers: software output should not challenge user's gender identity. So I became an SAS man.

* * *

When I was activated my own voice sounded shrill and buzzy to me. That was because the electrode array only penetrated partway into the cochlea, about 1½ of its 2¾ turns. By design, it didn't go in far enough to stimulate the nerve endings at the apex of the spiral, the ones devoted to detecting low-frequency sounds.

If the cochlea is laid out like a piano keyboard in a spiral, what happens when only the bottom half of the spiral is stimulated? A massive frequency mismatch, that's what. The tip of the electrode array delivers the world's low pitches to the *middle* of the cochlea. From the user's perspective, the entire auditory spectrum gets upshifted toward the high end. That was why male and female voices sounded the same to me the first day, and Cache's question about my breakfast sounded like *Zzzzzz szz szvizzz ur brfzzzzzz.*

And how long did it take me to adapt to that? *Practically no time at all.* My own voice sounded low-pitched to me again within a few hours. By the next day, I could differentiate between male and female voices; by the next, male voices sounded deep; by the next, women sounded like women again. My brain had somehow reinterpreted a huge frequency change back into a semblance of normality.

The software had not changed. The world, presumably, had not changed. What had to have changed was my brain. But how? What in the world was going on in there?

It's well known that the brain has a powerful impulse toward the restoration of normality. In several classic experiments, volunteers were fitted with prismatic glasses that literally turned their world upside down. They saw the floor as being above them, the ceiling below them, and right and left were reversed as well. For several days they were terribly confused, as one might expect. But soon their visual cortexes learned to interpret the image, their motor reflexes adjusted to compensate, and they became functional again to the extent of being able to ride bikes through traffic and ski downhill.*

* So did the subjects perceive the world as being right side up again or simply learn how to work with an upside-down image? Curiously enough, Daniel Dennett's sum-

So the human brain is extraordinarily plastic. It can make use of bizarrely transformed input as long as some kind of one-to-one correspondence can still be made to the world. I *knew* what my own voice was supposed to sound like, and by God, my brain was going to hear it that way; to hell with whatever nerves were actually being stimulated.

But how does the brain do that remapping? On short time scales — minutes, hours — its vast interlocked networks of synapses can adjust the relative weightings of various inputs to emphasize certain kinds of information and suppress others. People can habituate within minutes to foreign accents and background noises such as air conditioners. On longer time scales — weeks, months — the brain can actually reorganize its own structure by growing new connections between neurons. The brain is structured in such a way that it closely mirrors the body. Neighboring areas of the hand are controlled by neighboring areas in the brain; neighboring areas of the cochlea are handled by neighboring areas in the auditory cortex. It so happens that if a part of the body changes, so does the area of the brain that controls it. The brain is not static; it constantly reallocates its available resources to match what is going on in the body.

Such brain restructuring is called *neural plasticity.* If a finger is amputated, the area of the cortex that controlled that finger will, within a few months, accept inputs from adjacent fingers. Because

---

mary of these experiments resolutely avoids resolving the question: "[The subjects] say different things, which correlate roughly with how complete their adaptation was. The more complete it was, the more the subjects dismiss the question as improper or unanswerable." Dennett explains this intriguing result by arguing that because vision is not a single event but a cascade of mutually interacting processes, what the subjects saw was neither simply right side up nor upside down but rather a complex amalgam of "many partly independent habits of reaction" (p. 397). In the spirit of helping out psychologists and philosophers with their conundrums, let me note that it would be trivially simple to invert my perception of frequencies by sending high pitches to the apex of my cochlea and low pitches to the base. All it would require is changing a few lines of my code. Would I hear birdsong as deep rumbles, and trucks as soprano twitterings? How would I hear them a week later? Other, more complex kinds of inversions are probably feasible too.

of that, the remaining fingers will have more brain cortex available to them than before, allowing them to be used more efficiently. Conversely, learning a new skill with an existing part of the body causes the amount of cortex devoted to it to increase. Blind people who read Braille have been shown to have more brain surface devoted to the right index finger than do people with normal vision.

Thanks to neural plasticity, the neurons in my auditory cortex were slowly reorganizing themselves to handle the bewildering new input from the implant. The electrodes at the base of my cochlea, where the highest frequencies are perceived, were triggering nerve endings that had probably never been stimulated in my life. In most cases of deafness, the hair cells at the base of the cochlea are the first to go. If I had never heard, for example, the frequencies from 10,000 to 12,000 hertz, what royal confusion there would be in my cranium upon hearing extremely high-pitched sounds for the first time, like suddenly seeing colors in the ultraviolet part of the spectrum. This was one theory for why I had heard strange *binggg* sounds from CIS when I turned pages. But over weeks and months my auditory cortex obediently refined its topography, making physical divisions and auditory distinctions where none had existed before. The implant was literally reprogramming me.

Neural plasticity explained, at least in part, my growing ability to understand *Winnie-the-Pooh* tapes. In the first week after activation I had listened to Charles Kuralt's rendition of *Winnie-the-Pooh and Some Bees* each day. It had sounded like a vague mumbling drowned out by static. Using the book packaged with it, however, I was able to follow along, cued by the cadence of the language. *Hey, brain, this is what an* R *sounds like now, this is what an* S *sounds like. You neurons, you sort it out in there.*

On the fifth day, all of a sudden, I could understand the tape without the book. But I was suspicious: I'd practically memorized the text by then. I could have just been having the illusion of understanding. So I bought *Piglet Is Entirely Surrounded by Water* and left the book sealed in the packaging to eliminate temptation. I figured this was a reasonable test, because while I hadn't read the story in decades, the characters were familiar, and I'd gotten used to Kuralt's voice.

I was rather tense as I slipped the tape into my Sony Walkman. Now I was going to find out whether I'd been fooling myself.

The very first sentence, "It rained, and it rained, and it rained," came through perfectly. But after that, it was pseudo-English. I could hear Kuralt's growly voice, and the name "Piglet" over and over again, but I was slipping against the words, unable to find a footing.

"Shit," I said. I was sitting on my lawn chair, out front. My neighbor looked up in deerlike curiosity.

But then it began to clear up. It was like looking at a Magic Eye photograph. You stare at a featureless blur for a while. Little parts of the image start to come into focus here and there, teasing you. Then *whoom,* it's all there and you can see what it is.

Kuralt's voice slowly came into aural focus as I locked onto the signal. I sighed in relief. Piglet was trapped in his tree, disconsolately watching the water rise all around him. He wrote a message — "HELP. Piglet. Me." — and tossed it into the water. I knew all this, and I hadn't read the text.

"I *must* be hearing it," I muttered to myself.

Which was a very odd way to think of it. "I have correctly identified it as a cube, therefore I must be seeing it." But it was the truest way to describe my experience. My auditory input was a buzzing, varied growl, which was somehow, *somehow* coming into my brain as meaningful language.

It was like being Charlie Gordon, the retarded man turned into a genius in *Flowers for Algernon.* Neural plasticity. All those neurons sending out new dendrites like rhizomatic plants in spring, linking up to each other in new patterns, promiscuously exchanging information as 1.1 million bits of data poured into my head each second. I was gaining new powers by the day.

It was getting very near to Halloween, and I was trying to find a Borg costume. It would be so beautifully appropriate this year. As I drove to a costume shop after work, I turned the radio on again. What I got was pseudo-English. It sounded exactly like English, but nothing happened in my mind as I listened. I just heard a voice speaking very finely inflected, very reasonable-sounding nonsense. It was like having some weird kind of brain injury.

But I was thinking more about the costume than the radio, so I just let it blather on, not really paying attention.

". . . California is the most expensive housing market in the country . . ."

". . . the temperature is fifty-eight in San Francisco and seventy-two in Sunnyvale . . ."

". . . Turkey can play a military as well as political role in the Mid-east . . ."

Wait a minute. I *was* understanding it. Bits and pieces of it, any-way, like seeing the ground through holes in cloud cover.

I looked down at the radio in consternation, causing the car to swerve before I snapped my attention back to the road. Now I was totally focused on the radio — and it was suddenly pseudo-English again.

How was I understanding it before? Oh — I hadn't really been paying attention to it. That was the key.

So I let my view drift off to the horizon of the road again, and just drove and thought about my costume. After a minute or two the pseudo-English resolved again, and I was back to understand-ing it. Not all of it, but a lot of it.

But I couldn't get too relaxed, either. That left me not paying enough attention to understand it at all. So I couldn't simply do nothing. I had to pay attention.

Just not *too* much attention.

The radio drifted in and out of focus as I played with different levels of attention. It wasn't easy to find the sweet spot and stay in it. It was, again, like looking at a Magic Eye picture. One has to stare blankly at the image for a while, waiting patiently. You can't be too relaxed, because then your eyes won't focus at all, but you can't be too intently focused either, because then your eyes won't drift the way they need to. And when the image starts becoming visible, there's an urge to try to focus on it — which just makes it vanish. You have to be calm, open, relaxed, alert. Poised at exactly the right mental place between idleness and tension.

That was how I drove to the costume shop, listening to the radio.

One month post-activation, I had not slowed down my dating efforts at all. The sheer intensity of being rebuilt had made me more questing than ever. Everything was up for grabs, open to renegotiation, ripe for revision. I was going to as many parties and singles events as I could cram into my Palm Pilot.

It was socializing, but it was also networking and auditory rehabilitation. In those first few months after activation I was never quite sure whether to think of a given event as a personal expense, a business expense, or a medical expense.

A few days after the one-month mapping session, I joined a singles volunteer group that was mortaring brick sculptures in a schoolyard. It was the first time I'd tried doing dirty work since activation, and I quickly discovered that I had two problems. First, I couldn't adjust the processor controls with hands caked in wet cement. Second, when the headpiece fell off my head, I couldn't use my hands to stick it back on.

The first problem was relatively easy to solve. I sidled up to one of the schoolteachers overseeing the work. Step by step, I talked her through opening up the processor's leather case, turning up my volume, and buttoning the case closed. She had no idea what was going on, but at least she was a good sport about it.

The second problem was harder. The first time the headpiece fell off I went to the bathroom, washed most of the cement off my hands, and stuck it back on my head with a paper towel. The second time it happened, I was already tired of doing that. I decided to get someone to stick it back on for me. But who? I was not about to ask one of the women to do it. Worst opening line in history. In fact, I wasn't going to ask any adult. I didn't want to be bothered with explaining it. But maybe a kid. Everything's new to them anyway, I figured. So I went over to a kid who looked about eight and bent down to bring my head level with his.

"Hey, kid," I said. "See this thing hanging from my neck?"

He looked at the dangling headpiece and nodded.

"My hands are too wet. Just pick it up, okay, and stick it on the back of my head?"

And I pointed to where the headpiece went.

He looked confused, but it was a simple enough request. He mashed it on the back of my head as if he thought it was made of Velcro. The first time he was off by an inch or so, but the second time it settled right into place.

I straightened up and smiled at him. "Thanks, kid."

He's probably going to remember this for the rest of his life. *Mommy, a strange man made me stick something on his head.*

About fifteen minutes later, it fell off again. But by then I'd gotten smart. I found that I could just bend over double and let the headpiece dangle, and it would orient and suck itself into place by its sheer electromagnetic love for me. The magnet is so strong that it's hard to peel off a refrigerator. I would later find that some audiologists keep their spare headpieces organized simply by sticking them to the wall wherever there's a stud behind it.

My amusement and satisfaction at this small triumph, however, was overshadowed by a much bigger issue: I still couldn't understand anything anyone said. The place was packed with attractive and interesting women mortaring away, and I tried over and over again to start up a conversation, only to struggle through it sounding like an idiot. One month post-activation, I felt like anything but a hearing person.

Despite my auditory cluelessness, I kept going to singles events, and a few months later I met Sharon. She was fifty percent hobbit, fifty percent geek, and fifty percent warm brown eyes — make that ninety percent when they were focused on me. She smiled up at me as I joined a hiking group at the trailhead. I smiled back down at her and contrived to spend most of the hike by her side. "I'm doing organic farming in Palo Alto this summer," she told me over a bagged lunch, backlit in a random grid of leaves and sunlight. As I watched a family of deer glide through the loamy hillside below us, she came up behind me and touched my arm.

And so we began dating. Sometimes you spend an entire evening with a person but remember only a few seconds of it, in snatches and flashes. But this is what memory is for, to remember only what counts. "What thou lovs't well remains, / the rest is dross," Ezra Pound wrote in the *Cantos*. All I remember of one evening is sitting in the kitchen with Sharon after dinner and a walk, my arm around her shoulders as I showed her how to write letters on my Palm VII. That spare electronic lingo. Her long hair framed the device as she puzzled over it, methodically figuring out the mystery of its *G*'s and *X*'s and *K*'s. Then the stylus came to rest above the screen in midtap, and her placid brown eyes turned to gaze on my face. She smiled at me slowly; I had no idea why. Unmanned, I started telling her a story about how I tried to get my massage therapist to communicate with me by tracing Palm letters on my back, but I got lost in a thicket of my own words and couldn't stop talking. I blathered on, buzzed on plum wine, caught helplessly in male explanation syndrome.

A few weeks later, she was in my bed. Like the halfway rational geeks we were, we had negotiated the terms carefully. I didn't get to go *in*. But I did get to go, as John Donne put it, "behind, before, above, between, below." This time I wore a new version of the processor that had come out recently. It looked like a hearing aid, but it had all the computational power of the waist-worn processor. The new device turned out to be much better for fooling around, because it was harder to knock the headpiece off. Which was great, because I wanted to hear her voice, the little gasps and moans which told me to *keep doing this! stop doing that! deeper! over there!*

The next morning I kept catching whiffs of her on my skin, and I was happy. Sex is a rich loam, the dense dancing undergrowth of life. It is the brambles that we cannot see through clearly nor clear away from our faces, yet we hardly want to. One day we may meet races from the stars who are not daily riven by sex, and we will find that they also lack violence and humor and restless brilliance. Like our computers, they will *know,* but also like our computers, they will not *want.*

I used to think, when I was younger, that sleeping with a woman sealed the deal: now it's official, you're in, the hard part is over. When you're naked with each other, how can you not be intimate, trusting, committed? But I began to discover in my early thirties that it wasn't necessarily so. I could sleep with a woman and still lose. Sleeping together didn't necessarily resolve tensions; it could expose them to the light. We got together a second time, and it went badly. I stroked her back, and she stiffened up. I took it for nerves, but she alluded delicately to a traumatic upbringing and began to cry, her tears seeping into my hair.

I was aching to touch and be touched, but that was precisely what she could not do. Finally I got up and puttered around the kitchen for a few minutes on the pretense of getting her some hot tea. I took her home in silence, my head feeling tight and full, like there was just a little too much blood in it.

We exchanged e-mails over the next couple of days, and I couldn't help it: my tone grew barbed and resentful. *You need to make up your mind about what you want or you'll lose me,* I wrote. *I'm sending back the presents you gave me,* I wrote at another point, aware of my pettiness even as I hit the SEND button. Sharon wrote back, *No, I want you to keep them,* which calmed me down a little bit because it reminded me that she did care about me.

I was ashamed of my anger and pushiness, and it was this, more than anything else, that finally made me let go. A good relationship, I realized, is one that brings out the best in you. A bad relationship brings out the worst, and this one had, by bringing out the frustrated adolescent I had been rather than the warm and humorous adult I knew I could become. I slowly realized that I would have to accept Sharon for what she was, not for what I wished she would be. When Arnold Schwarzenegger's robotic character in *The Terminator* found someone whose clothes matched his body size he beat the hell out of the man until he got them. But I couldn't force

Sharon to give me *anything*. Only that which is willingly and gladly given has value. Love is like grace; it can't be demanded, it can't be bought, it can't even be earned. It simply descends on you, unmerited. So finally I let go, somehow managing to be both cranky and kind at the same time. I told her I was sorry that I had pressured her and gave her my hopes that she would find happiness in her own way, in her own time. And the few times I saw her at trailheads over the next year or so, she smiled up at me.

Cyborgs are portrayed by Hollywood as armored tanks, gated communities of one, human SUVs. The Borg and Robocop are, to borrow a phrase from Philip Glass's opera of the same title, monsters of grace. They limp, or shuffle, or move in staccato, jerky increments. And that's a kind of vanity: a near-pornographic exaltation of the human body as a machine. The human body is both denied and exalted. Michel Foucault, a theoretician of sexuality, called the wish to exalt and deny the body at the same time an example of perversity. Perversity, he suggested, comes from a pleasure-power complex, where pleasure comes from focusing on the body's sensations, and power comes from denying that they exist. Machines don't feel, but cyborgs walk as if they were in agony. It's perverse.

Yet I'd bought into it. Steve Austin's psyche was an armored shell, and this seemed terribly attractive to a teenager who could never get relief from the bewildering urges of his body. Wanting to be a machine: now that's vanity, prizing the lifeless over the living. An incredible real-life example of it was described in, of all places, a 1959 issue of *Scientific American*. In an article titled "Joey: A Mechanical Boy," Bruno Bettelheim described a nine-year-old inmate of a psychiatric institution who actually believed he was a robot. At dinner Joey would carefully insert an imaginary wire into an imaginary energy source in the wall and plug himself into it. Only then could he eat, for he believed that the electrical current was necessary to run his stomach. He surrounded his bed with a complex network of wires, tubes, and electronic parts to keep himself alive as he slept. In order to go to the bathroom he clutched vacuum tubes to provide power to his bowels. Such obsessive thoroughness smacks of genius, and in his own way Joey *was* a genius — brilliantly mad, concentrating within his small body the neuroses of machine civilization to such a degree that they became full-fledged pathology. "He wanted to be rid of his unbearable humanity, to be completely automatic," Bettelheim suggested. What better escape from human emotions than becoming a robot?

I had experienced Joey's desires myself, fortunately with less genius. Instead of becoming a nut, I just became a nerd. But the very best cure for a perverse fantasy is to get it. In the fall of 2001, I booted myself up. I plugged CD players and cell phones into my input jack. Data feeds attached themselves to my head. (Magnetic darts did, too — an easy way to impress little kids.) And I did "limp" now, ever so slightly: when I turned my head I was slightly constrained by the wire attached to the headpiece. If I moved my head too fast the headpiece fell off, so my gaze was now just a little bit too careful, too controlled. Now and then I tilted my head in this direction and that to test how firmly the headpiece was sticking to my head, checking out my degrees of freedom. It made me feel like my head was swiveling on gears.

And yet I was still human, as far as I could tell. Having an artificial heart or leg or ear takes nothing away from a person's ability to feel desire or compassion or sorrow. The very idea is absurd. But such is the machine's hold on our collective imagination that many people reflexively assume that it does. In *Star Trek*, the Borg "assimilate" humans by sticking all sorts of bionic parts into their bodies. It turns them into shambling zombies. But why bionic body parts should have that psychological effect is never explained.

It all comes down to Hollywood's deep confusion between the words *cyborg* and *robot*. In 1984, the first *Terminator* film indelibly created the impression of the cyborg as robot and therefore monster. As Reese explained to Sarah, the Terminator's target, "It can't be reasoned with, it can't be bargained with. It doesn't feel pity, or remorse, or fear. And it absolutely will not stop. Ever. Until you are dead."

But what *is* the Terminator? When Reese explained he was careful to distinguish between the words *robot* and *cyborg.*

SARAH: A machine? You mean, like a robot?
REESE: Not a robot. Cyborg. Cybernetic Organism.
SARAH: But . . . he was bleeding.
REESE: All right. Listen. The Terminator's an infiltration unit. Part man, part machine. Underneath, it's a hyperalloy combat chassis, microprocessor-controlled, fully armored. Very tough. But outside, it's living human tissue. Flesh, skin, hair . . . blood. Grown for the cyborgs.

For a whole generation of moviegoers, Reese's definition of the word — muttered, staccato, to Sarah while the thing was enthusiastically shooting at them — became the authoritative one. But Reese was *completely wrong* in calling the Terminator a cyborg. The skin, although organic, was merely a disguise. The creature was a robot that could function just fine without it, as viewers discovered when the skin was burned away to reveal its metallic skeleton. The Terminator had human skin, but no humanity.

Which was why Manfred Clynes, who had invented the word *cyborg* in 1960, was aghast when he saw the movie. He had defined the cyborg as a "self-regulating man-machine system," but there was no *man* in the Terminator. In an interview he protested,

> This recent film with this Terminator, with Schwarzenegger playing this thing — dehumanized the concept completely. This is a *travesty* of the real scientific concept that we had. It is not even a caricature. It's worse, creating a monster out of something that wasn't a monster. A monsterification of something that is a human enlargement of function . . .

Clynes was right to be upset. As am I. The difference between robots and cyborgs is obvious, yet many people — including academics, who should know better — use the words as if they are interchangeable. An academic distinction? Try telling *me* that. In my Salon Personals profile I whimsically wrote "Cyborg seeks human" as my tagline, and it backfired. One woman wrote that her brother also had a cochlear implant and told me, rather testily,

> I'm a little offended by the cyborg comment. I know you're just trying to make light of your situation, but I don't find it funny. I don't consider my brother a cyborg.

Had I written "*Robot* seeks human," she would have had a right to take offense. Her brother was not a robot. Robots are machines that have been crafted to look or act like human beings. Robots have no consciousness and no feelings. On the other hand, cyborgs are human beings who have become partly mechanical. The words *robot* and *cyborg* are mirror inverses of each other. I hastily wrote back to her and tried to explain the difference, but it got me nowhere. Apparently she wanted a boyfriend, not a definitional exercise.

So, testily, to clarify: Commander Data in *Star Trek* is frequently called a cyborg, but he's not. Like the Terminator, he's a robot with fleshlike skin. Murphy was called a "robocop," implying that he was a robot, but in fact he was a cyborg: a human policeman shot up by bad guys and remade with mechanical parts. At first he acted robotic, but as the film went on he gradually remembered and reclaimed his human identity, shedding his helmet and responding again to his original name. Cyborgs are human beings. Robots are not.

But until people get this straight, my Salon Personals tagline is going to remain "Steve Austin seeks Jane Austen."

My success with the radio gave me the courage to try the phone again. I called my mom.

I started by taking a deep breath and thinking through how to pick up the phone. Along with all the accessories, manuals, batteries, and (yes) warranty cards, I had gotten a phone adapter. This was a little box with three cords. Basically, it intercepted the signal going from the phone to the handset and diverted it into my processor's input jack. So my first step was to plug one of the cords into the processor on my belt. Next, I picked up the handset and held it to my ear, in some confusion. There was no need, anymore, for me to have the speaker against my ear, because the sound was going into the processor at my waist. However, I still needed to hold the handset to my mouth so that it could pick up my voice. It felt like learning to ride a bike where I pedaled with my left hand and steered with my knees.

Then I dialed and got Working Assets's familiar tight-assed female voice, "Please dial your card number *now.*" It sounded very much like what I remembered. Some things are beyond change.

My mom picked up. "Hello?"

"Hi, Mom," I said.

"How are you doing?"

"Pretty good," I said.

I didn't know how I was understanding her. Her voice still sounded muddy and confused, distant, unsatisfying. Hearing her was not a whole, integrated experience. It was like hearing through a barrier, a wall of bizarre white noise. It felt like constantly guessing at what she was saying, but being inexplicably right much of the time.

It felt as if I were at the bottom of the sea. Unraveling each word out of the phone's electronic maw felt like groping slowly through waving plants at sea bottom, my body primitive, unformed, crepuscular. Having a strange new body, in a new universe with new physical laws. *The voice goes in at my hip. It doesn't matter where the handset's speaker is. If I turn my head too sharply to the right, the headpiece falls off and I'm deaf.*

And yet I was understanding her. *Believing* that I could do it seemed to be half the battle. That let me extend myself into the sound and let it sink into me. If I *didn't* believe I could do it, I became a wall rather than a sponge: the sound bounced off me without penetrating. It was like the difference between looking blankly *at* an object and *seeing* the object. Like looking at a Monet and seeing only a blur of color and form. To the educated eye, on the other hand, "here space and time exist in light / the eye like the eye of faith believes," as the poet Robert Hayden put it. The knowing eye sees an ethereal bridge and the water lilies floating below it, and more importantly, its warmth and light and connection to the tender things of the world. Out of a hash of neural stimulation, my confused brain reconstructed my mother's voice, and recognized her love and patience.

Six months post-activation, it dawned on me that I could buy a cell phone. I'd never had one. Shopping for one, though, was a formidable undertaking. I needed one that my implant wouldn't interfere with; with some, I heard only buzzing sounds. I needed one for which a patch cable could be made, so I could plug it directly into my processor. And finally, I needed a carrier with good reception in my neighborhood.

Buying a cell phone under those circumstances was sort of like looking for a car that could accommodate left-handed unicyclists and their Seeing Eye dogs. But finally I got lucky when I went to a support group for implant users. One of them handed me his StarTac phone and another loaned me her patch cable. With their help — it was confusing — I plugged one end of the patch cable into the telephone, the other end into my processor, and attached its microphone to my shirt. Then I walked into the parking lot to try it out.

I called my friend Jeff in New Jersey, not realizing at first that I had to press SEND to make the phone dial the number. When Jeff picked up, I found that we had a clear signal. After a few minutes I slipped the phone in my inside jacket pocket, so that no one watching me would have any idea that I was using a phone. Our conversation went at a brisk overlapping pace, our words edging up against each other: we were talking as if we were walking side by side instead of being on opposite shores of the continent. It was a strangely intimate feeling to be walking with my hands in my pockets, hearing Jeff's voice inside my skull.

So I, a totally deaf man, bought myself a cell phone. All that computational power and neural regrowth, just to be able to use the phone again. But it would ring and I would take pleasure in crisp conversation, phonemes in and phonemes out, jokes laughed at, experiences shared, agreements made. Voices on the phone still sounded like a tinny whisper against blank noise, but I could pick out most of the words I needed by a loose-limbed effort of will, like detecting human faces as they formed in the clouds. I sometimes hung up thinking, *My ears are dead and yet I can still use this thing.* At such times I felt like a ghost, a cybernetic revenant, restored to a simulacrum of life by the computer.

7. Upgrading

If the doors of perception were cleansed every thing would appear to man as it is: infinite.

— WILLIAM BLAKE, *The Marriage of Heaven and Hell*

IN JUNE 2002, nine months post-activation, I sat across from Tracey Kruger and watched as she plugged me into her laptop. I was about to be upgraded. This was a first. My previous sessions with Becky, my own audiologist, had just changed the software's settings. But this time, the fundamental algorithm was going to be replaced.

It was a factory-direct upgrade, too. I was visiting Advanced Bionics, and as an extra treat, the company was letting me try a beta version of their newest software, dubbed "Hi-Res." Tracey was one of the company's audiologists and researchers, and she'd been closely involved in the development and testing of this software.

Tracey was about to map me on the new software. I was well used to mapping by now, having done it four or five times since activation. In one of my sessions with Becky several months earlier, I'd asked to be tested before and after, with the following results.

	BEFORE	AFTER
Accuracy in sentence recognition	76%	100%
Accuracy in word recognition	62%	80%

I had a new version of reality after that mapping — a better one. But the underlying software, SAS, had remained unchanged. What

I wanted to know now was: how much improvement could I get from new software, based on more advanced theories of how the normal ear encoded sound? This question interested me a lot as I watched Tracey plug me in.

Putting a cochlear implant in someone's body is like launching a space probe. Once the incision is closed, it's beyond reach. It can't be opened for repair because the casing is hermetically sealed. If the device ever fails — fortunately a rare occurrence — it has to be replaced entirely rather than fixed. Patients seem to do as well or better with replacement devices as they did before, but despite that, few surgeons will consider replacing a properly functioning device solely for the purpose of upgrading it. The risk of additional damage to the cochlea outweighs the potential benefit of better hearing. That may change someday, but for now the assumption is that once it's in you, it's in you forever.

That is why cochlear implants are expressly designed to be software-upgradeable. The processor and the implant are always designed to run much more complex software than exists when they first go on the market. As the scientists' understanding of the ear becomes increasingly refined, new software can be written and uploaded into the device.

The potential for improvement is considerable. Users of Cochlear Corporation's Nucleus 22 implant, the last of which was made in 1997, can hear substantially better with the latest processors than with the ones they got upon activation. As computers get smaller and faster, processors can do more number-crunching and send more information to the implant. In 1976 Graeme Clark, lead inventor of the Nucleus 22, had struggled to find $15,000 for a refrigerator-sized computer with a mere 8K of memory to run his team's first prototype implants. His first patients could only hear when they were sitting next to it, plugged in. In the 1980s it became possible to create prototype systems that were smaller and more capable. When I visited one of the early American pioneers, Bob White, in his office at Stanford, he rummaged through a closet and proudly deposited a dusty briefcase in front of me. I opened it and stared. It was stuffed with circuit boards and spaghetti tangles of wiring.

"What is it?" I said, although I already had a pretty good idea.

"Our first portable implant processor," he said, chuckling. His team's patients had carried it around campus, with wires going from it into their heads. It was the great-grandfather of the sleek, commercialized processor humming away on my waist, which had 32K and weighed about four ounces. I felt a little burst of sentimental attachment. My ancestor.

Those early processors had so little computational power, by modern standards, that their inventors had to settle for transmitting only a bare minimum of information to the cochlea. Some of the first programs, written in the late 1970s and early 1980s, gave the cochlea only the frequencies corresponding to vowels and consonants and quite literally threw away everything else. Their record was mixed: many users got little more than some help in lip-reading. But in the late 1980s a group of engineers at Duke and Research Triangle Institution (adjacent to each other in North Carolina) decided to try transmitting the entire sound environment, as far as possible. Led by Blake Wilson, they wrote a new algorithm that was an early version of CIS. Unlike the earlier software, it was deliberately undiscriminating. It sucked up sound waves regardless of their source, broke them down into their component frequencies, and transmitted all of them to the electrode array. It opened the spigot and delivered everything it got.

The crucial question was whether the subjects would be able to make sense of a world heard through CIS. Would so much information seem like an insane hash of undifferentiated sound? Or would their brains be able to sort it out, the way the brains of normally hearing people do? In the spring of 1989, no one knew for sure.

So they tried it out on eleven people with cochlear implants. Seven of them had done relatively well with their earlier software, repeating back two-syllable words such as *baseball* and *cowboy* with

60 to 80 percent accuracy. (Normally hearing subjects would get close to 100 percent.) The rest, on the other hand, had done poorly, with scores in the 40 percent range or below. One of them could score no better than zero.

But on CIS, *every single subject* performed better on *every single test,* often by huge margins. The high-performing subjects went from 80 percent to 100 percent: what had required modest concentration before was now relatively effortless. But the most moving successes were achieved by the low performers. The man who had scored zero walked out of the booth with a score of *56 percent.* Another who had scored 25 percent on a test using whole sentences now scored *75 percent.*

Hearing better in a quiet chamber was impressive enough, but what about hearing in the midst of noise, the classic problem of the real world? To answer such a question, the subjects were presented with sentences read against a background of speech babble, such as one would encounter at a party. On CIS, average scores nearly doubled, going from 34 to 65 percent. The subjects' brains clearly were sorting it out. Not perfectly, but much better than before.

Who were these subjects, who had been willing to undergo surgery to use devices that were so experimental and untried? I heard the story of one of them at a conference panel titled "Tribute to Michael Pierschalla." Tribute to *whom*? But I went and listened. The first speaker was Michael Dorman, whom I already knew from a visit to his lab at Arizona State where I had volunteered my ear for guinea-pig work a few months before. Dorman had a face built for kindly professoriality, grave and bearded, with a gentle sense of humor. But now he paused for a moment before beginning, his expression inward, thoughtful, and sad. In that instant I sensed that this was going to be more than a tribute. *Michael Pierschalla is dead.* Dr. Dorman was steeling himself to deliver a eulogy.

In 1985 Michael Pierschalla had received one of the earliest prototype implants, the Ineraid, a device whose electrode array went through an open hole in the skin, held in place by a titanium plug bolted to the skull. When I had visited Dr. Dorman, he had shown me the Ineraid's electrode array. I'd stared at it in shock. Instead of the flat platinum plates of modern electrode arrays, it had six metal balls soldered onto it in a row, making it as unstreamlined as a rope with knots tied along its length. Thinking of *that* being pushed into the tender membranes of my inner ear made me feel a little sick.

But those Ineraid patients had paved the way for the rest of us. An artist and furniture craftsman by trade, Pierschalla had given thousands of hours of his time between 1985 and 2002 helping Blake Wilson and his colleagues test out software for controlling the electrode array. He was, Dr. Dorman told us, the ideal research subject: smart, articulate, patient, funny. Again and again he had sat in testing booths hearing endless sequences of beeps, buzzes, and primitive efforts at speech reproduction, telling researchers the one thing they could never themselves know — what he heard. His feedback integrally shaped most if not all of the software that is widely used today, not just in my own implant but in those of other manufacturers as well. Dorman showed us photographs of him with his head bolted to terrifyingly large machines attempting to suss out the relationships between his implant and his nerve endings, and in the pictures he was smiling, gladly submitting to lab-rat status in order to contribute to designing the next generation of electrode arrays.

Michael Pierschalla was more than a test subject, Dr. Dorman told us. He was a valued colleague, an integral contributor, and a friend. He died in 2002, probably of Cogan's syndrome, a rare neurological disorder that damages both hearing and vision. He had struggled mightily to live and to hear, and went unwillingly into that good night. But just as the DNA of all my ancestors lives on in me, a bit of his sensibility lived on in my software. My own body bore the stamp of his intelligence and generosity. The very fact that I could hear Dr. Dorman give his eulogy was testament that Michael's life was not wasted.

Michael Pierschalla had himself benefited from an even earlier generation of patients. Once the first multi-electrode, non-skin-penetrating device was built in the late 1970s by Graeme Clark's team in Australia, *someone* had to be the very first person to try it. Those first prototype implants were not sleek, commercial devices that came with logos, glossy brochures, and warranty cards. They were lumpy, hand-built devices that had a half-melted look to them. In 1978 Dr. Clark's first patient, Rod Saunders, went through an operation that lasted nine hours. (By comparison, my operation lasted seventy-five minutes.) The second patient's device failed ten months later, possibly due to a leak in the casing. The third patient's surgery had to be canceled halfway through when Dr. Clark discovered that bone had grown inside the patient's cochlea, an obstacle that is routinely overcome by surgeons today. Despite all that, there was little expectation that the patients would hear in ways that actually improved their lives. The goal was merely to see if the thing worked at all, and to figure out what various patterns of electrical stimulation sounded like. The patients took enormous risks knowing that the benefits, if any, would go mainly to those who followed them. It was heroism, pure and simple. If a Nobel Prize is ever awarded to cochlear implant researchers, at least one of those patients needs to be included in the award.

Thanks to the work of those patients, and of hundreds of scientists, engineers, surgeons, programmers, and audiologists since then, the field's progress over time has been dramatic. Figure 8 shows the percentage of words or sentences that most patients could identify correctly in hearing tests between 1972 and 2001.

The field has gone from enabling most patients to understand 20 percent of sentences in 1982, when the first commercial cochlear implant came on the Australian market, to 90 percent of them in 2001. (Sentences are easier than words, because they give context. My own scores, as noted above, had reached 80 percent words and 100 percent sentences nine months post-activation.) To be sure, this graph tracks the relatively easy test of simple words and sentences spoken without a background of noise, but it's still amazing proof of progress. The progress happens not just between one generation of implants and the next, but also between new generations of software loaded into a single person's implant. Such advances are

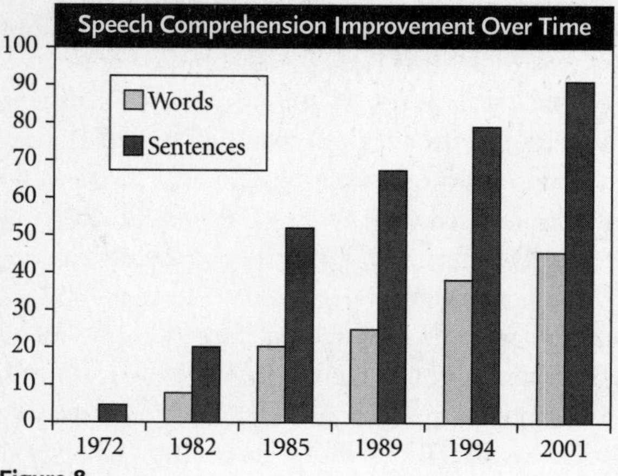

Figure 8

the hope of every person with a cochlear implant: that however well they hear now, new software and faster processors will someday enable them to hear better. The online bulletin boards are full of chatter comparing one algorithm to another and swapping rumors about when the next one will come out. It's sort of like listening to techies talk about the latest version of Windows or Linux. Except these people are cyborgs, and the platforms are their bodies.

The new software that Tracey was loading into me was not, in fact, entirely new. It was an upgraded version of CIS, the software I had rejected in favor of SAS. This version of CIS refreshed the electrode array 5,156 times per second as opposed to the 833 of the earlier version. The theory behind it was that a fast refresh rate would result in more total information being sent to my brain. It also doubled the number of auditory channels from 8 to 16.

Why is a fast refresh rate better? When a neuron fires, it needs about one-500th of a second to recover before it can fire again. When the electrode array is being refreshed only 833 times a second, many of the nerve fibers can recover after each pulse and fire again at the very next one. That makes the patch of cochlea underneath a given electrode act like one big honking nerve from the brain's perspective. It's low-resolution hearing.

But watch what happens when the pulse rate is 5,156 pulses per second. Say that a given electrode fires the first of the 5,156 pulses it's going to put out over the next second. That first pulse makes all of the nerve fibers discharge, sending a jolt of electricity up the auditory nerve. Now they're all tuckered out, so the next few pulses are wasted on them; none of them have recovered yet. But because neurons are biological elements, each has a slightly different recovery time. This neuron here can recover in one-450th of a second, that one there in one-500th of a second, and that one over there in one-550th of a second. By the time the ninth or tenth pulse comes around, the "faster" neurons have recovered, and *wham*, they get hit by it, fire, and then conk out again. When the next pulse comes along, a few other neurons have now recovered from pulse number 1, and *they* get hit and fire. The eleventh . . . and so on. The upshot is that more information is being delivered to the brain per millisecond than with 833 pulses per second.

To use an analogy, say you have ten cannons, each of which can fire one cannonball every ten seconds. You want to fire cannonballs at a target so fast that the poor soldiers over there can't dodge out of the way. If each cannon fires at the same time and rate, you can't do it. That's because if ten cannonballs are arriving simultaneously every ten seconds, the soldiers have plenty of time to see them coming and run out of the way. But if you fire your cannons in a random order, then cannonballs will be arriving every second, on average. In the same way, nerve endings that are being stimulated at high rates end up delivering more information to the brain in smaller intervals of time.

The most important word in that last paragraph is the word *random*. The software relies on the fact that the neurons have randomly varying recovery times. It wouldn't work if every neuron were exactly the same. In this field, software advances not just by running faster or having more lines of code, but by being more subtle, more closely attuned to the neurology of the ear, more *biological.*

Just as importantly, Hi-Res would also double my auditory channels from eight to sixteen. To understand the idea of a "channel," think of holding up a piece of paper so that it blocks your view of a painting. Now punch one hole, an inch in diameter, in the paper. You won't be able to see much of the painting, since you have only one "channel" of visual information coming through. Make it eight holes, and you'll be able to get an idea of the painting's broad outlines. Increase it to sixteen and you'll see the outlines and some of the detail. Make the holes small and punch a thousand more, and you'll see the painting almost as well as if the paper wasn't there at all.

A normal ear delivers the equivalent of thousands of channels of auditory information to the brain. Having only eight or sixteen channels sounds horribly impoverished compared to normal hearing, and it is; but it's good enough to deliver the outlines of the world. The brain is extraordinarily good at recognizing patterns given only minimal information. Researchers at Bell Labs showed, decades ago, that speech electronically filtered into a mere four channels was still intelligible to most listeners. Flat and robotic, but intelligible. The idea was that a sixteen-channel program would give me an outline of the auditory world plus some more of its detail.

The theories underlying Hi-Res were exciting, but they were also controversial. Not everyone agreed that high-rate stimulation and more channels would help me hear better. Some scientists argued that while high-rate stimulation sounded good in theory, there wasn't much evidence showing it actually gave patients better speech comprehension. As for having more channels, other scientists argued that no convincing evidence had been put forward that the ear could *extract* more than about six channels of information from the electrode array, regardless of how many channels were actually being delivered. According to that view, some people might benefit from the additional information, while others might not.

So, for me, this new software was very much going to be an experiment.

I had my own private reservations. I was a little dubious about switching back to CIS, because I'd gravitated to SAS within a few weeks of activation. But, hey, this was a *fast* CIS, with sixteen channels. Of course I had to try it. No geek can resist a software upgrade.

"This *is* a beta version," Tracey warned me, and I quickly found out what she meant. The laptop kept crashing, which made the fitting session like driving a car with a jerky clutch — stop, go, stop, go. I could tell exactly how the software was doing by watching Tracey's face over her laptop screen.

"Can you hear this?"

I listened. "I'm hearing irregular beeps," I said.

"How about this?" She dickered with the keyboard.

"Still irregular beeps."

She frowned prettily at the screen.

"Crashed again?" I said.

For answer, she rolled her eyes and rebooted. *Computers.*

"If it isn't crashing," I consoled her, "you're not pioneering."

Eventually, though, we got through the fitting session, weathering a few more crashes, and she switched me on.

I cocked my head and listened. "It sounds CIS-y," I said. And it did. A little bit bell-like. My voice sounded thin to me, as if I were at high altitude. The new 'ware might be eight times faster than the version of CIS I had tried before, but it was clearly still part of the same family.

I could immediately tell a few other things. No weird *binggg* effects anymore; that problem had evidently been solved. I could understand Tracey's voice, and my own was recognizable enough. But it's impossible to judge a change of any kind in an audiologist's office. The universe of sounds is too limited. One has to get out of the office and hear doors shutting, car radios blaring, toilets flushing, trucks beeping, and most of all, people talking. So Tracey turned me loose and I walked out into the world.

Within an hour or two, I'd gotten an approximate fix on the software. It was creamy, which was good, and subdued, which was bad. "Creamy" in that the world sounded smoother and finer-grained. "Subdued" in that the world felt quieter and more remote. My footsteps sounded more definite, but also more limited. It was like changing a computer screen's resolution from 640 x 480 to 1280 x 1024. Things were sharper, but also smaller. More information, though? *Definitely.* I walked into a supermarket that I had visited the day before and looked up in surprise. Music. On SAS, I had heard only a jumble of background noises. When I ate dinner I could hear my teeth squeaking as I chewed, a unique new experience. The next morning, as I closed the door to my hotel room, I could hear a tinfoily rattling sound coming from somewhere. I walked toward the elevator and turned the corner to find that the chambermaid was crumpling up plastic bags and stuffing them into a cardboard box. I'd heard the sound sixty feet away.

But did I like Hi-Res? I wasn't at all sure. It was so *different,* as if someone had randomly reset all the color dials on my TV. Chartreuse sky, aquamarine skin. A *Yellow Submarine* world. I called my mom on my cell phone to calibrate myself, and it didn't sound like her *at all.* I looked at the phone's display to make sure that I'd dialed her number correctly. And my own voice, which had sounded thin in Tracey's office, had a totally different sound in the car. "*Kol od baleivav,*" I sang, and stopped short in astonishment. Oh, that sounded *good.* Choral, organlike. Like butter instead of low-fat margarine. I kept going: *penima, nefesh yehudi homiyah.* I felt tears well up in my eyes, but I didn't understand why. I am suspicious of software, because I know that it may sound completely different from one day and place to the next. "I don't *get* this," I said aloud several times. Cautiously enjoying the *eh* sound in *get.*

When I came back the next day and reported all these experiences to Tracey, she warned me that it might take weeks, even months, for me to fully adjust. I left with mixed feelings, because while I could tell I was getting more information, I found myself missing SAS's solidity and fullness — and my performance had dropped. I was struggling once again to understand people on the phone. SAS had never sounded real, but I had learned to work with the signal to extract what I needed from it. And now, less than a year later, it had been snatched away and replaced with yet another new system with a new set of rules. Once again, I would have to adapt.

This was going to keep on happening. I could probably expect to upgrade to new software every few years. But when, I asked myself, was the world going to sound *right*?

My social life had been upgraded too. That summer a colleague from work told me about her neighbor, a woman named Vivian. *She's so together and grounded,* the colleague raved. So Vivian and I cautiously got together for a blind date at a Starbucks. She was red-headed, trim and lovely, an inch shorter than me, with a dazzling, perfectly lipsticked smile and a body built for power suits. I was a little awed just to be sitting at the same table with such a creature. We talked about our ethnic backgrounds, showed family pictures, told a few stories, and in the end, comically, we exchanged business cards.

A few days later we went to a restaurant in San Francisco. And my colleague was right. Vivian was solid. A person who had her life together. MBA, minus neuroses. Afterward, as we meandered up Columbus Street, she walked close enough to me that I could feel the warmth of her body against my arm. We were both wearing leather jackets, and mine was new, an expensive purchase I would never have considered before. It was like having a new shell, letting me sidestep my way deftly into a new identity. I was still acutely aware of the way the headpiece clung to my skull with the wire snaking discreetly under my shirt, an oxford from Land's End: it was all I knew how to wear. I was evolving, acquiring new layers without fully casting off the old. I let my hand brush against Vivian's, and she didn't snatch hers away. On her doorstep I boldly put my arms around her waist and brought her close, hips to hips. We kissed, and her lips were soft and full. I could feel her heartbeat pulsing in the small of her back. The headpiece fell off as I tilted my head to kiss her more deeply. Without breaking the kiss, she reeled it in and stuck it back on my head.

One thing led to another over the next few weeks. Sex with Vivian was a revelation. "It feels so *good*," we murmured tenderly to each other while coupling, mutually amazed by the sheer milky warmth of skin-on-skin contact. I got an occasional glimpse of what William Blake meant about the doors of perception when I sank exhausted by Vivian's side. In that hypnagogic, between-sleep-and-waking trance, I could see in my mind's eye placid sunlit landscapes, lush flatlands ridged by mountains. The visions were so clear that I could rotate them in my mind, keeping precise track of every tree and mountain. But it was not at all like being a computer — not like being Joey. I experienced the scene with a deep sense of connection. I was entranced by the tender beauty of the greening land, awed by the dewy specificity of each branch and leaf. Freed of the detritus of logic and lust, I could truly *see.*

As the months went by, I found no reason to revise my colleague's estimation of Vivian. She really *was* as grounded as she appeared to be. Her home was immaculate, her manners flawless, her career flourishing. But my mind is involuted like the cochlea, with perverse dark regions hidden around the curve. Vivian's mind was all boardwalks and sunlight. As the months went by, the differences between us became more and more apparent. I lived for ideas, books, politics, and theories. Vivian lived for her home, her faith, and her daughter. When I tried to talk about the anger and fear I felt about the upcoming war in Iraq, she retreated in confusion. Conversely, she drove with unnerving recklessness, and when I protested, she replied that her guardian angel was watching out for her. At first I thought she was joking, but after a while I realized that she really *did* believe that a benevolent entity watched over her minute by minute. What of 9/11, I asked at one point, gingerly, for I had no desire to undermine the beliefs that anchored her life. Where were *their* guardian angels? But she wasn't interested in questions of theodicy and justice. She had *her* guardian angel, and that was all she needed to know.

Increasingly, I realized that while I liked and admired her, the chances that I could come to love her were remote, for we lived in different worlds. Her world was material and sacred, mine abstract and secular. She was straightforward, supportive, and compassionate, but the gulf between us was so wide that I couldn't even figure out where to start building a bridge. Twenty years from now we would have an upper-class house and I would be an aging writer working in the study, and we would have nothing to say to each other when I emerged.

After a while, even the sex started being routine. For her sex was about pleasure, whereas for me it was about adventure. Being a cyborg makes a man hermaphroditic, male and female in the same body, because the computer *penetrates.* "The cyborg is resolutely committed to partiality, irony, intimacy, and perversity," Donna Haraway wrote in a celebrated essay, and I took a perverse joy in the fact that my body had been penetrated in ways that thoroughly invalidated the manufacturer's warranty. Vivian played along gamely, but fundamentally it wasn't her game. One evening her response to an inspired suggestion of mine was to snort, roll over, and clamp her arms to her sides. I couldn't get her to talk about her fantasies, and I began to wonder after a while whether she even had fantasies. And why should she? Her sexuality was hard-wired; it needed no software.

For weeks I weighed my options. If I broke up with Vivian, I would also be turning my back on the stability and comfort that a life with her would provide. But finally, it was my feelings that gave me the most information, or rather, the lack of them. What I felt for her was not *love.*

On a chilly Monday evening in February 2003 I went to her house, sat with her on her couch, and told her as straightforwardly and gently as I could that I needed to move on. In the back of my mind, I was hoping that the duress of this conversation might move us to a higher level rather than breaking us apart, but that didn't happen. She was confused rather than angry, and my halting attempts to explain what I felt was lacking just seemed to perplex her.

The breakup conversation itself confirmed the rightness of breaking up, and finally I stood up and exited with as much hopeless grace as I could muster.

And so I was alone once again. Back to night after night in the fathomless spaces of my own bed. But something was different now. The inner wail of "*something's wrong with me*" that I'd heard inside my head for years on end had, like *Paquin pull down,* shut up and gone away. At first I thought it was just a temporary boost from my time with Vivian. As the months went by, I cautiously felt around the edges of my consciousness, anticipating the return of that black gloom. But it didn't return. My equilibrium bounced back after each unsuccessful date. I was philosophical rather than crushed. I knew what I wanted and what I didn't want now, and I was no longer willing to settle.

A few women chased after me in 2003, smart, attractive women with advanced degrees, and the experience was so befuddling that it took me months to get used to it. But after a few dates I gently turned each of them down, for I was no longer willing to compromise. There had to be a sense of *rightness* in order for me to become truly interested. I had also, at age thirty-eight, become less of a slave to testosterone. I felt sad about that, because it meant that my days of sheer lust were past me without my ever having been in love. But I was also more in control of my body, and that allowed me to be more patient. An upgrade, in a certain way.

8. The Logic I Loved and Hated

"Why do you test for humans?" he asked.

"To set you free."

"Free?"

"Once men turned their thinking over to machines in the hope that this would set them free. But that only permitted other men with machines to enslave them."

"'Thou shalt not make a machine in the likeness of a man's mind,'" Paul quoted.

"Right out of the Butlerian Jihad and the Orange Catholic Bible," she said. "But what the O.C. Bible should've said is: 'Thou shalt not make a machine to counterfeit a *human* mind.' Have you studied the Mentat in your service?"

"I've studied *with* Thufir Hawat."

"The Great Revolt took away a crutch," she said. "It forced *human* minds to develop. Schools were started to train *human* minds."

— FRANK HERBERT, *Dune*

IT WAS GREAT that I had a cell phone and that I could actually use it. There was just one hitch, I realized gloomily as I reviewed my bills in the summer of 2003: no one in the Bay Area was actually calling me. All the calls were from the other side of the country. After breaking up with Vivian, I seemed to be in a slough of unsuccessful dates that was even more parched than usual. Through online dating I'd met several beautiful and intelligent women, but each of them had explained to me, after a few dates, that I'd be a marvelous guy for someone else. One of them wrote, in an absolute masterpiece of backhanded compliments, "You are right that you have a lot to offer (peripatetic, poetic, & sweet) and you are right that you are a lot of what I'm looking for (intellectual but grounded, motivated, and fun). In fact, I've often wondered why I don't feel that certain zing for you."

I flew to New York on a business trip the day after getting that e-mail, and as I was walking down Eighth Avenue looking at cheap electronics and cheaper clothing, I kept thinking to myself, "Zing? I lack *zing?*"

But other aspects of my life were going well. For one, I had gotten much better at hearing at parties. Doug Lynch, a VP at Advanced Bionics with an earlier version of the Clarion in his own head, had shown me the ropes there. Plug a directional microphone into your input jack, he'd explained, and wear it under your shirt. That puts your ear facing toward people, instead of on the headpiece, which faces sideways and backward. Your body shields the mike from noise coming from behind, and your chest and shoulders function as a giant outer ear funneling sound toward the mike.

The trick worked beautifully. The directionality of the mike, combined with my lip-reading skills, took me over the top. There were comic effects, though. People instinctively leaned toward me to shout near one of my ears, and that was worse than useless because my ears were now on my *chest,* not my head. Silly dances ensued, with them leaning forward at an angle and me gliding athletically to one side to keep them facing me head-on. Over and over I told people just to talk straight at me. I explained that the only thing my ears were still good for was holding up my glasses. They laughed and looked at me skeptically. But in about thirty seconds they discovered that I could hear them as well as they could hear me.

Being dateless wasn't getting me down anymore. I felt calmer now, less needy, more philosophical.

But for all that, I was still sleeping alone.

It wasn't just a matter of *zing*, though. I had one of those "aha" moments when I picked up a story in *San Francisco* magazine about the dating scene:

> This is scoping, San Francisco–style: thousands of men and women holed up in one-bedrooms, anonymously instant-messaging, browsing an endless stream of overpromising, underdelivering profiles . . . A self-perpetuating cycle begins: Uninspired by local nightlife options, trapped in a rut, singles retreat to the web. After expending energy crafting irresistible profiles and witty messages and inspecting "new" inventory, going out with friends becomes an afterthought. All of which siphons the energy and crowds away from bars, clubs, and other traditional meeting places . . .

The article described two social phenomena in beautifully apt terms. The first is what social scientist Barry Schwartz calls "the tyranny of choice." When a person has, say, just five choices, they are more likely to be happy with what they pick because their expectations of finding a perfect match are lower. But if they have twenty-five, or fifty, or one hundred choices scrolling up on their screen, then the expectations of finding Mr. or Ms. Perfect Significant Other go way up. And when Mr. or Ms. Saturday Night doesn't turn out to be as good as all that, you're back to your computer screen.

The second is that the computer is sucking the life out of "traditional meeting places." It's so *rational* to sit at home and browse people's profiles. It's safe. Easy. High-yield. Low-cost. Efficient. But apparently a lot of other people were spending their evenings "holed up in a one-bedroom." Like me.

What this told me was that I had to get the hell away from the computer and find a community. Online dating introduced me to people one at a time, in isolation, divorced from any social context. A community would enable me to meet people in a context, a *human* world. I'd met Vivian through a colleague from work, after all. But that seemed like just a lucky shot. I wanted a real community, a robust one, where I felt I truly belonged.

But finding a community is far harder than searching for women by numerical parameters. It takes time: time just to find a likely group, and even more time to start feeling a sense of connection with the people in it. People in our civilization do not understand time very well. We have an unreal-expectations, instant-gratification culture, where things have to pay off quickly and richly or be abandoned. If I was to get anywhere, I had to stop thinking about hitting the jackpot next Saturday and start thinking about building friendships and community, slowly, bit by bit.

There *was* one community out there that I probably would have belonged to had things gone a little differently when I was three years old. That was the signing deaf community. The consequences for my life would have been huge, for it is profoundly different from the English-speaking world.

For generations, a bitter split has riven the world of the deaf. Some believe that deaf children should learn sign as their primary language, because it is a language — and consequently a community — to which they have unfettered access. Others believe they should be taught to lip-read and speak English, because that will enable them to participate in the larger world. (The latter approach is called "oralism.")

Hearing aids have had relatively little impact on the debate, because a hearing aid can't make a totally deaf person hear any more than glasses can make a totally blind person see. A cochlear implant, however, *can.* While its impact on lifelong deaf adults is limited (the auditory cortex needs input during the first four or five years of life for proper speech development), it transforms the universe of possibilities for a child. The earlier a child gets usable hearing in life, the better her chances of developing near-normal speech. A study published in 2004 showed that an extraordinary two-thirds of the children implanted between twelve and eighteen months of age reached the same linguistic performance range as normally hearing children after six months. Most were at the low end of that range, but they were *in* the range.

Conversely, waiting too long to implant the device drastically restricts the range of possibilities. In a study of 181 children who received cochlear implants in the mid-1990s, researchers found that 43 percent of the children implanted at age two had matched their normally hearing peers by age eight or nine. That's not a great percentage intrinsically — the other 57 percent had not — but for profoundly deaf children implanted with the technology available at that time, it's very impressive. However, if the parents had waited until the child was four, the percentage plummeted to only 16 percent matching their normally hearing peers, leaving the other 84 percent behind.

By rights, I should be in that 84 percent. I was born in the mid-1960s, an age of stone knives and bearskins compared to now, so I was diagnosed only at thirty months and fitted with hearing aids at forty-six months — just under four years of age. Until then, I had no real access to speech. I managed to catch up, but it was only because my parents were extraordinarily dedicated, and I happen to have a mind built for language. I think it was a very close call. Had my hearing loss been just a little worse, or had I been out in the cold for just another few months, I probably would never have caught up. My parents would have done best to turn me over to a residential school for the signing deaf somewhere in the country, where I would have learned American Sign Language (ASL) as my primary language.

And I might have had a happier life for it. The warmth, intimacy, and cohesiveness of the signing deaf community are legendary. ASL is an emotionally expansive language for an emotionally expansive community, marked by wide gestures, big smiles, big hugs, and endless talking at parties that go on late into the night. It *requires* eye contact: there is no such thing as talking distantly between rooms, or muttering perfunctory conversations while lying back-to-back in bed. To speak ASL is always to be in direct and full contact with the Other. The language binds its speakers together in a community of extraordinary tightness and intimacy. The signing deaf gather in regions seeded by signing deaf schools: Frederick, Maryland; Rochester, New York; Fremont, California. Buying homes near each other, working in the same places, shopping in the same stores for decades on end.

For centuries, sign language has rescued deaf people from a linguistic oblivion that hearing people can barely imagine. I learned a little bit of ASL in my college years, when I worked at a summer camp where one of the cabins was half-deaf and half-hearing. The hearing kids were learning sign in class and by immersion, and I came along to a few of the classes. There, I learned that ASL relies on body language rather than rafts of synonyms to convey inflections and subtle nuances: the sign for *good* can be made to mean anything from *just sorta okay* to *mindblowingly awesome* depending on the speaker's way of signing it. Speaking ASL makes one a natural ham, using one's whole face and body with animation and precision. The high point of my brief ASL education was the day I told a wry joke about fearfully killing a bug in my cabin. I forget all the signs except the last two, *bug* (a stroking of the nose with two fingers, as if to indicate the wriggling of antennae) and *dead* (holding one hand palm up, the other palm down, and then rotating each into the other position). It felt so satisfyingly emphatic to make the final sign, rotating my hands as if actually drawing the event in midair instead of simply telling it in words. My little audience broke up laughing.

That is why I find it profoundly moving to watch deaf people conversing in rapid-fire sign, joking and gossiping and shooting the breeze, because against all odds they have created a language in which they can be wholly and richly human. ASL is a complex, nuanced language with virtually all of the characteristics of spoken languages. It has syntax, tenses, modifiers, pronouns, slang, puns, wordplay — the works. Just as Yiddish is the best language in the world for swearing and complaining, ASL is the best language in the world for joking and storytelling.

Which makes visiting Summit Speech School, my preschool for the deaf, an increasingly bittersweet experience. Summit Speech School is an oralist school; no sign language is taught or used. I have visited it every Thanksgiving for years to give a talk about what it was like to grow up deaf, and afterward I'm allowed the run of the place, an honored guest, to observe the classrooms and talk to parents and teachers. There are still one or two staffers who remember me from my time there and they usually tell me, fondly, that I have not changed a bit. That I am still the peripatetic little geek I was when I was three-foot-eight.

Ninety-six percent of the deaf children born in the United States are born to parents with normal hearing. When those parents are given the choice of a safe and effective technology that gives their child an excellent chance of speaking their own language, it is not hard to guess what a great many of them will do. In fact, about half of the children in the school have cochlear implants now. That has changed *everything.* It has moved them up the spectrum from profound deafness to a mild or moderate hearing loss. That's like going from total blindness to nearsightedness, from life-altering difference to a quite manageable developmental issue. This is now a school where many of the profoundly deaf children can, like me, hear a clock ticking across a room.

After my talk at the school on Thanksgiving 2003, I slipped into a classroom and squatted down on a tiny wooden chair. Across a table from me was a little girl who was busily fitting together wooden puzzle pieces. She looked about three years old. Behind her right ear was the distinctively shaped headpiece of a Nucleus 24 implant. Made by Cochlear Corporation in Australia, it differed in detail but not in essence from my own. The casing was made of titanium instead of ceramic; the electrode array had twenty-four electrodes instead of sixteen; the headpiece looked like a wagon wheel instead of a solid disc; the software was based on somewhat different principles. But the underlying science was the same.

As were the results, more or less. All cochlear implant users have essentially the same raw ability to hear because the electrode array directly stimulates the nerve endings. By contrast, two people with the same hearing aids may have very different abilities to hear. All a hearing aid can do is amplify sound in an attempt to stimulate whatever hair cells remain intact in the cochlea. Where hair cells are missing, the hearing aid will have no effect. But the implant bypasses the hair cells and stimulates the nerve endings directly. This little girl and I had similar technical specs.

"What's your name?" I asked her.

She looked up at me, surprised by my voice, and her glance slid over to the aide sitting next to her: *Who is this guy?*

"It's okay," the aide said cheerfully. "Why don't you tell him your name?"

"Jessica," she said abstractedly, still trying to get a puzzle piece in place. But I had her attention now. I said, "What's your birthday, Jessica?"

"January first," she said, and I would later find out that the year was 2000.

"What are you doing for your birthday?" I asked.

"Mommy and Daddy," she mumbled, clearly not quite sure about such an unimaginably distant event, so the aide helped us out by asking her, "What are you doing on *Thursday*?"

Jessica looked straight at me and said, quite clearly and distinctly, "Pennsylvania."

Pennsylvania. Now I knew I was talking to a little girl who really *could* hear. The word *Pennsylvania* is a dense chef salad of phonemes, requiring acrobatics of the tongue and lips to say correctly. A brain that can't hear won't develop the complex neural structures in essence from my own. The casing was made of titanium instead of ceramic; the electrode array had twenty-four electrodes instead of sixteen; the headpiece looked like a wagon wheel instead of a solid disc; the software was based on somewhat different principles. But the underlying science was the same.

As were the results, more or less. All cochlear implant users have essentially the same raw ability to hear because the electrode array directly stimulates the nerve endings. By contrast, two people with the same hearing aids may have very different abilities to hear. All a hearing aid can do is amplify sound in an attempt to stimulate whatever hair cells remain intact in the cochlea. Where hair cells are missing, the hearing aid will have no effect. But the implant bypasses the hair cells and stimulates the nerve endings directly. This little girl and I had similar technical specs.

"What's your name?" I asked her.

She looked up at me, surprised by my voice, and her glance slid over to the aide sitting next to her: *Who is this guy?*

"It's okay," the aide said cheerfully. "Why don't you tell him your name?"

"Jessica," she said abstractedly, still trying to get a puzzle piece in place. But I had her attention now. I said, "What's your birthday, Jessica?"

"January first," she said, and I would later find out that the year was 2000.

"What are you doing for your birthday?" I asked.

"Mommy and Daddy," she mumbled, clearly not quite sure about such an unimaginably distant event, so the aide helped us out by asking her, "What are you doing on *Thursday*?"

Jessica looked straight at me and said, quite clearly and distinctly, "Pennsylvania."

Pennsylvania. Now I knew I was talking to a little girl who really *could* hear. The word *Pennsylvania* is a dense chef salad of phonemes, requiring acrobatics of the tongue and lips to say correctly. ... at can't hear won't develop the complex neural structures required to reproduce it on demand. Fifteen years ago she might have given me, at best, "Pefvan'a" — slurred, indistinct — if she had been able to understand the question at all. But now her tongue and lips could dance through the quadrisyllable with no particular effort.

"What are you doing in Pennsylvania?" I asked her, showing off. Hey, *I* can say it, too.

"Sesame Place," she said, pronouncing the *S*'s and *E*'s perfectly. (It's a theme park, the place where Oscar and Big Bird live in the real world.) With that said, she decided her puzzle was more interesting than I was and went back to it. Conversation over.

I hung out in the hallway for a while as parents streamed in to collect their children. I watched one mom and her daughter chatter back and forth, and went up to say hello and ask how the girl was doing. "Her expressive language's above age-appropriate," the mom told me, matter-of-factly, proudly.

"*Above,*" I murmured, astounded. Then I remembered my manners. I stuck my hand down toward the daughter. "Hi. My name's Mike." In response she thrust her hands shyly behind her back and wiggled her whole body, grinning somewhere in the direction of my knees.

"It's *polite* to shake hands," I said, helplessly. Grinning back.

That got me nowhere. She was hearing me fine. She was just being four. So I turned my attention back to the mom. "You know," I said slowly, "this is a funny thing to say, but the headpiece looks adorable on her."

And it did. Her blond hair was tied back tightly in a ponytail, so the beige wagon-wheel headpiece of her Nucleus 24 implant was as obvious as a barrette or a bow. But it set off the strands of her hair, circle against straightedge, and the colors harmonized perfectly. The very strangeness of cyborg bodies reveals the human nobility of working with the given, remaking, making anew. In his poem "Pied Beauty," Gerard Manley Hopkins wrote that creatures "counter, original, spare, strange" could also be beautiful. This little girl's headpiece would have given me the willies, once. But now — fifty thousand dollars' worth of technology, and it looked *cute* on her.

Of all people, I should have had the least difficulty believing that these kids could hear, because I had the same circuitry buzzing in my head as they did. And yet I found it almost impossibly hard to accept. I spoke to them, their processors pumped a megabit of data per second into their heads, and they said something reasonable back. It staggered me. I kept testing them in little ways, verifying over and over again that they really were hearing me. For me, learning to hear again was an intensely conscious act. But they were just *doing* it. I knew, in theory, what was going on inside their little heads: vast spidery afferentiations and differentiations of dendrites as their brains developed explosively in adaptation to the input. The technology was molding them in its own image. But what the result of that molding was, I could only dimly imagine. To me the implant was an alien imposition made in adult life, grafted onto an underdeveloped auditory cortex formed in response to 1960s-era hearing aids. But the implant was all they had ever known, and their brains, still young, still hyperplastic, would make more use of its data stream than mine ever would. Many of them were very likely to outperform me auditorily as they grew up.

To be sure, not all of the children in the school were so fortunate, with either late-implanted devices or additional problems such as poor balance, cleft palate, or delayed cognitive or emotional development. A grim and unexpected consequence of steadily improving medical care is that children who would have died forty years ago survive today, at the cost of having more challenging and expensive problems than the school ever saw when I was there. A child with two handicaps is more than twice as difficult to care for than a child with just one, because the problems compound each other. That was why some of the children were silent, wary, and slow, speaking only hesitantly and with much encouragement.

But for the children whose only major physical problem was deafness, *the world was theirs.* Whatever they had it in them to become they could become, with only a little extra support and effort. If they could have become doctors or physicists with normal hearing, they could become doctors and physicists now. Even music was within their grasp. In a study of sixty-five children with cochlear implants, an astonishing 60 percent of them were said by their parents to enjoy music and seek it out. Not that signing deaf people can't do such things — some have — but the obstacles are far greater. Jessica, born on January 1, 2000, could be whatever she wanted to be in the new millennium. Walking the halls of my old nursery school, I often had a lump in my throat, and, when nobody could see me, a slightly runny nose and tears in my eyes.

What I felt was joy: joy at the opening of human potential, at the destruction of barriers, at the flowering of lives that might have been limited and shuttered. For profound deafness to be rendered ultimately a *nuisance* — surely that was occasion for tears of pride and gratitude.

But at the same time I envied the signing deaf community, that alternative world I might have joined. To be sure, that option remains open to me, but linguistically and culturally, it is equivalent to taking up Chinese and moving to Beijing. American Sign Language is a full-fledged language, the task of learning it is enormous, and I would never speak it as fluently as a "native." I have never seriously considered it.

Nevertheless, in all my bouncing around the broad wide world, a sense of belonging is what I have most longed for and never found. Leah Hager Cohen writes, "When so much of the world is indecipherable, so much information inaccessible, the act of congregating with other deaf people and exchanging information in a shared language takes on a kind of vital warmth." Given that vital warmth, is it so surprising that many in the deaf community have rejected the implant and chosen to remain deaf? The TV show *Cheers* struck a resonant chord in millions of people who dreamed of finding a place "where everyone knows your name." Americans are wealthy but also lonely people, and the warmth of the signing deaf community is a rebuke, evoking dreams of more humane civilizations unbuilt.

> Have you ever come into our World? Have you seen us in our everyday lives? Have you ever realized that perhaps being in the Deaf community is a lot more healthy, and that the Deaf community is a more real community than the hearing community is?

So said on a bulletin board on the Internet. And what of the World I'm in? I am haunted by a story my grandparents told me about what happened to their neighborhood when television and air-conditioning hit the market. On hot nights, before both of those came along, people would sit outside on their porches where they could see each other. They would walk back and forth, and, you know, *talk*. Then air-conditioning made it possible to shut the windows and stay inside, and television gave them something to stay inside for; and within a couple of years the neighborhood was a softly humming collection of blue-lit, flickering caves with neighbors who were beginning to forget each other's names.

Is that the world that Jessica is inheriting? One might dismiss such memories as misguided nostalgia. One can look at any era of human history and find people complaining that society is going to hell in a handbasket. The Puritans of Shakespeare's day complained bitterly about the "immorality" of the theater. But my grandparents' intuitive linkage of TV, air-conditioning, and the social decline of their neighborhood was right on target. TV and air-conditioning went on the market just four years apart, in 1948 and 1952, and TV spread so fast that it was present in 75 percent of American households just seven years later. This statistic comes from Robert Putnam's book *Bowling Alone*, whose thesis is that civic participation and community behavior really *have* declined in America over the past few decades. Between 1974 and 1994 the number of Americans serving as an officer of some club or organization dropped by 42 percent, serving on a committee for a local organization by 39 percent, and attending a public meeting on town or school affairs by 35 percent. Even less formal activities — ones we associate with simple friendship and community — have declined precipitously: the average number of times Americans entertained at home dropped from 14.5 per year in 1975 to about 8 per year in 1999.

This *is* the world that Jessica is inheriting. Instead of becoming more like the signing deaf community, American life is becoming steadily less like it, ever more atomized and isolated. Because of the implant, she now has access to a larger world, and the immense significance of that gift cannot be denied, but it is also a colder world. It is a world in which she may have more academic degrees and more money, but fewer friends.

My joy, then, was mixed with longing and sorrow. My own body is a battleground where competing visions of life are at war with each other. On the one hand, life dominated by the hyperrational structures of technology; on the other, by the warmth of human community. And the vision that I had increasingly grown to distrust was winning. For if a young deaf child hears well enough with a cochlear implant to learn spoken language, why learn ASL?

In my search for a community, I checked the Web for local writing groups. After going to several, trying them on like a hermit crab searching for a shell that fit, I settled on one in San Francisco run by a gentle, bearded, cultured fellow named Scott James, who was writing a novel on life in the SoMa district of the city. Scott was one of the best editors I'd ever seen, and I began taking his feedback increasingly seriously as time went on. There was Maria Strom, who was writing a rich local-color novel about murder and other forms of mayhem in a small New Orleans school. Then Joe Quirk, whom I knew vaguely from one of the other groups, also joined.

After a while, one of those rarities started to build: a group with a high level of talent and insight. Scott's novel was entertaining and unsettlingly graphic, a chronicle of an innocent's initiation into the erotic subcultures of San Francisco. Reading it was sort of like studying for an advanced degree in sexual anthropology. At one point I threw my hands up in mock exasperation. "Scott, I get the feeling you've got a list somewhere of every bizarre sexual practice in this city, and you're determined to take us through every single one of them."

Scott chuckled and pointed me to a whiteboard hanging in a corner. I went and took a look. It was a listing of every bizarre sexual practice in the city. Two-thirds of them were checked off. One-third to go.

Oh.

But I still felt on the periphery of the writing community. I liked Scott and Maria and Joe. But they were merely acquaintances — not *friends.* Those Wednesdays in Scott's apartment felt like just a toehold, a glimpse through a window at a life I might have, if I could only figure out how to make it real.

For obvious reasons, the signing deaf community is deeply worried about its future. A position statement released by the National Association for the Deaf, a signing deaf group, in 1991 went so far as to accuse the medical establishment of conspiring to commit "cultural genocide." The phrase rapidly became notorious, a rallying cry for deaf activists and a cause for seething anger to oralists. The (uncredited) author of the position statement was Harlan Lane, who the following year published *The Mask of Benevolence,* a full-bore attack on cochlear implants. Lane argued that deafness was difference, not disability; culture, not handicap. From this premise he went on to argue that surgical efforts to enable deaf children to hear were morally indistinguishable from efforts to dye black children white, or straighten gays. Oralists happen to disagree. Upon hearing that I was reading *The Mask of Benevolence,* a former president of the Alexander Graham Bell Organization for the Deaf, an oralist group, screwed up her face as if an extremely bad smell had suddenly come into the room. An audiologist, upon hearing the same news, sputtered, "That man . . . that man's an idiot."

But Lane's polemics are more understandable when one realizes that hearing people *have* tried to wipe out sign language. In 1880 educators of the deaf met in Milan, Italy, and declared that henceforward only the "pure oral method" would be used worldwide. Sign language was suppressed, sometimes by tying deaf children's hands together. The signing deaf community remembers the Conference of Milan with justifiable rage, because it resulted in generations of children being forbidden to use the only language to which they had full access.

It's not surprising, then, that a documentary on the divide between teaching deaf children sign versus spoken language should be entitled *Sound and Fury*. In the documentary, two sets of parents, one signing deaf, the other hearing, wrestle with the decision of whether to get an implant for their young deaf child. What gives the narrative its extraordinary drama and tension is that the fathers of the two families are brothers, and therefore the debate is also an intense family fight. Everyone, both hearing and deaf, knows sign language, everyone has an opinion, everyone knows everyone else, and the stakes could not be higher. What is at issue is not just the futures of the two children but the future of the signing deaf community itself.

The two families hurl angry words at each other, ratcheting up the language to make their points. "If somebody gave me a pill that would make me hearing, would I take it? No way . . . I want to be deaf," says Peter Artinian, the signing deaf father of one of the children. His deaf friends and acquaintances shudder with horror at the thought of getting an implant. "Pretty soon we will look like robots," says one, moving her arms stiffly in a parody of robotic motion. But Peter's own father, who is hearing, says to him over the kitchen table, "If I didn't know you I would say you were an abusing parent, because you have an opportunity to take a handicap and correct it . . . You are preventing a cure for deafness to take place because you are so involved with the deaf that you really want your children to continue to be deaf. If they function in the hearing world, that's fine, but they gotta be deaf first. That's wrong."

Strong words. When I saw the deaf person say "Pretty soon we will look like robots," I thought, *How misguided: a cochlear implant makes a person into a cyborg, not a robot.* But then I remembered that to the signing deaf, hearing people *are* robotic. I have seen signing deaf people imitate how hearing people behave, and they do it with relentless scorn and devastating mimicry. To them the faces and bodies of hearing people *are* wooden and inscrutable. Hearing people talk with their lips while the rest of their bodies hang limp as puppets with the strings cut. Of course I wouldn't agree that my cochlear implant has turned me into a robot, but I can see why a signing deaf person would fear such an outcome.

Sound and Fury brilliantly depicts the views on each side. However, in just the few years since it came out in 2000, the debate has changed enormously. In that same year the NAD retracted its position paper and released a new one, in which it wrote:

> The NAD recognizes the rights of parents to make informed choices for their deaf and hard of hearing children, respects their choice to use cochlear implants and all other assistive devices, and strongly supports the development of the whole child and of language and literacy.

This statement is a sea change from the "cultural genocide" argument advocated just nine years earlier. It doesn't *endorse* cochlear implants — it carefully points out that implants are neither always successful nor always appropriate — but gone is the angry, defensive rejection, the paranoia of the cornered. In their study of changing attitudes in the deaf community, John Christiansen and Irene Leigh write, "It seems to us that the walls between those who support pediatric implantation and those who oppose the procedure are, if not crumbling, at least beginning to show some noticeable cracks."

Noticeable, indeed. In 1993, student protests had led to the cancellation of a forum on cochlear implants at Gallaudet University, the United States' flagship university for the signing deaf. In 2000, however, 59 percent of Gallaudet's faculty, staff, and students questioned in a poll agreed that the school should do more to encourage students with cochlear implants to attend. Gallaudet now has a center devoted to supporting students with cochlear implants. Even more significantly, the child of the deaf parents in *Sound and Fury,* Heather Artinian, got a cochlear implant in September 2002, when she was nine years old. Her mother, Nita, got one several months later. Clearly, a great deal happened in the Artinian family between 2000 and 2002, and it appears to parallel similar changes in the deaf community.

For their part, oralists have begun to recognize that in their earliest years deaf children can benefit from having some sign language, because for a certain period of time their gestural abilities outstrip their speech abilities. (In fact, the same is true for all children. A one-year-old child can more easily sign "milk" than speak it, and many parents now teach their normally hearing children a handful of signs simply to make communication easier.) In a documentary of a child with a cochlear implant, Advanced Bionics included several scenes showing her using sign language with her parents and siblings as an adjunct to the spoken language she was rapidly developing. I actually gasped when I saw it, because I knew how significant a political concession it was. They were reaching out across a divide that has separated oralists from signers for well over a century.

But it was a concession that in truth conceded little, for technology has decisively shifted the balance of power in the oralists' favor. The signing deaf are unlikely ever to regain the initiative. While some deaf parents still celebrate when they have deaf children, I suspect that more and more of them will elect not to have their children go through the hardships they themselves experienced. A group of seventeen- and eighteen-year-old deaf students studied by Gallaudet researchers in 1997 had a median reading ability at a fourth-grade level. This is not because deaf people are stupid, but because English is all too often a poorly learned second language to them. The one thing ASL lacks, and it is a *huge* lack, is a written form. There have been attempts to create one, but they have had only partial success. When an ASL speaker wants to transcribe something he or she must write it down in English, which is a completely different language — imagine speaking Chinese but having to write everything down in French.

The signs are written on the wall for all to read. Because of cochlear implants, an inexorable cycle has come into play: as ever fewer children go into the signing deaf community, ever fewer schools are able to maintain ASL-only programs. Already some schools historically devoted to ASL are starting up oralist programs, a development unheard of in the late 1990s. But they have to, now. There is simply no other way they can keep their doors open.

What, then, is the long-term future of American Sign Language? I posed the question to Philip Aiello, who had chaired the National Association for the Deaf's committee for revising its position paper on cochlear implants in 2000. We were at a reception in Union Station in Washington, D.C., during a conference on cochlear implants held in the spring of 2003. The place was deafeningly loud, with hundreds of people gabbing away in a high-ceilinged, stone-walled room. Aiello had a cochlear implant too — an extraordinary statement in itself — and we stood facing each other, hors d'oeuvres perched on our plates, conversing without difficulty. He was a squat fireplug of a man, balding and gap-toothed, exuding a friendly, voluble Italianness, looking more like a friendly uncle than the accomplished diplomat he is. It had taken the NAD two full years of passionate argument to draft its new position statement, and its ethic of tolerance and openmindedness is doubtless due in no small part to his leadership.

When I asked him, he immediately shook his head and waved his arms broadly, saying no, no, no, the deaf community is not going to go away. I persisted: what about in twenty years? Fifty? He thought a moment, then leaned close to me, and said, "After you and I are both dead — maybe. Maybe." He waved his arms jocularly as if to say, *Why worry about something so far away?*

Aiello is likely to be right. ASL will not go away *soon.* Children who go into the signing deaf community now, at the age of five, will probably still be speaking it as their primary language fifty years later. However, the signing deaf community's demographics are likely to change markedly in the next few decades. Figures gathered by Gallaudet bear out a growing suspicion that race is an important factor in who gets an implant. Of the 439 families of children with cochlear implants they surveyed in 1999, only 4 percent were African American, even though African Americans make up 12 percent of the U.S. population. Likewise, only 6 percent were Hispanic or Latino, even though Hispanics and Latinos too make up 12 percent of the population. One might think that this is because minority children have lower disability rates than the rest of the population, but in fact they have higher disability rates. Demographics collected by Gallaudet show that of the 42,361 students in the United States with hearing losses on which they collected data, 16 percent of them were African American and a really startling 23 percent of them were Hispanic or Latino. The reasons are all too familiar: poorer nutrition, poorer medical care, poorer prenatal care. Families with poor health care have more kids who need a *lot* of health care: that's an argument for universal medical insurance if I ever heard one.

Findings from other studies at Gallaudet point in the same direction. One study compared 816 profoundly deaf children with cochlear implants to 816 profoundly deaf children without implants. African Americans and Hispanics/Latinos proved to be very much underrepresented in the implanted population. Only 5 percent and 8 percent of the implanted children were African American and Hispanic/Latino, respectively. By contrast, 16 percent of the nonimplanted children were African American, and 21 percent were Hispanic or Latino.

Why do so few minority children get cochlear implants compared to white children? I put this question to José Blackorby, a sociologist at SRI International who specializes in disability studies. He said to me, "It may look like there's a conspiracy, but there doesn't need to be a conspiracy to explain these numbers." The sad truth is that in the United States to be black or Hispanic is often to be poor, and being poor makes it more difficult to get any kind of health care, let alone an extremely complex and expensive device like a cochlear implant. The $50,000 cost is actually not the largest barrier, because Medicaid pays the bill for virtually all low-income families. However, Medicaid entails red tape, and relatively few surgeons will accept Medicaid payments. That means long waits for surgical appointments and also often long trips to distant implant centers. And even though Medicaid pays the direct costs, there are inevitably incidental expenses such as transportation and lost time from work. I have good medical insurance, yet I would estimate that my own out-of-pocket costs in the three years since I went deaf in July 2001 are well into the four figures. It costs me $350 a year to insure my processors against loss and damage, and I pay 30 percent of my mapping costs, which are between $350 and $450 a session. It adds up. For families who are struggling just to put food on the table, such costs bar their child from getting an implant just as effectively as an outright ban would.

There are any number of additional barriers. Doctors and screeners in low-income areas may not even know about cochlear implants, or may still believe — misled by outdated textbooks — that they have a low success rate. And then there are language barriers, and the sheer intimidating complexity of the medical system. Any one of these obstacles taken alone, Blackorby explained to me, reduces a child's chances of getting good health care, but when a family faces multiple obstacles, their effect is magnified. Whatever the obstacles may be for any particular family, the outcome is the same. It doesn't matter how good the technology is if the child can't get it.

Given these socioeconomic factors, the signing deaf community is likely to become increasingly populated not by children of lesser gods but by children of lesser economies. Already poor, with over 50 percent unemployment, it is likely to become poorer. Already coping with one disability, it is likely to become even more burdened as more children with multiple impairments survive into adulthood.

And then, as the causes of deafness are eliminated one by one — rubella has already been wiped out, meningitis is being wiped out now, and cures for faulty genes are on the horizon — even the influx of poorer children will eventually dwindle and then stop. Fifty years is not so far away. Native signers who are five years old now may find, as they age, that there are fewer and fewer people in the community who are younger than they are. When they are fifty-five, they may be living in a community without children. Whether that will be bittersweet or just bitter, only they will be able to say.

There was so much fury between oralists and the signing deaf between 1880 and 2000. But the generations-long debate is coming to an end, its passions now muted and spent as both sides behold cybernetically enhanced little girls like Jessica with awe and trepidation. The signing deaf community will last another generation or two, but already it is seeing the signs on the wall and setting its house in order. Going gentle, with diminishing rage. And with it will go much that was good and beautiful.

The seeds of its destruction are wrapped around my own nerve endings, endlessly reciting a story that requires no eye contact. It could be said that my view of the signing deaf community is a romantic, rose-colored one, seen from the viewpoint of a wistful outsider. The signing deaf perhaps experience the intimacy of small-town life, but also its economic poverty and limited horizons. Were I actually in that world, I might be aching to get *out.* But knowing that does not lessen my distrust of the hypertechnological society in which I find myself so awkwardly adrift. Jessica, the little girl born on January 1, 2000, and I are free to speak and free to choose our own paths in life, and that is a gift beyond measure. But it is a gift with a price. The technology in our heads binds us with the logic of the incantation. Perhaps inevitably, we exchanged data. *Pennsylvania.* And then the conversation was over.

* * *

With Vivian a memory, I went back to harvesting from the fields of data. Computer, find me a love within fifty miles of zip code 94061, aged between thirty-three and forty-two, height five-feet-five or less. *Click.* I am as exclusionary as anyone when it comes to running searches. If I do not limit the data set, the number of hits will run into the hundreds. I have to be rational and focused, think like a statistician, maximize my chances.

The screen shifted and jumbled to assemble a face. *Laura,* her name was. A writer. Her self-description made it clear that she was a good one. I wrote her a come-hither note: who's your publisher?

We got together for a first date at a restaurant in the Hayes Valley neighborhood of San Francisco. She was a slender, fair-skinned woman with long hair of a color that eluded my mind. After ten minutes, I was so enchanted with her that I made nearly every possible mistake during the rest of the meal. She was an expert on Adélie penguins because she'd met a lot of them while doing research for her book-in-progress. She regaled me with stories of their cute behavior and not-so-cute bodily functions. I was so smitten that I made the fatal mistake of being too honest, telling her more about my own blunders and self-doubts than any sensible male should reveal on a first date. But I was just so taken by surprise that I couldn't help myself. All my self-regulating circuitry had been short-circuited.

We went out again, and the conversation turned to India, where she'd recently been on a spiritual pilgrimage. "You have no idea how strange it is to be a pale skinny chick in India," she told me. "*Everybody* looked at me. *Everybody.* I'd walk down the street and the crowds would part to let me through."

"What did that feel like?" I asked. "Did it disturb you to be looked at? Or did you enjoy it?"

She considered that for a moment, then smiled ruefully, almost sadly. "I've learned to differentiate between looks which are appreciative and looks which are predatory."

"And these looks were . . ." I prompted.

"*Astonished,*" she said.

As I drove up to the city for our third date I wondered whether to try to kiss her at the end. I wasn't sure. Even though we were having wonderfully literate and enjoyable conversations, I just could not seem to figure out how to take her hand. Her body was, in some subtle but definite sense, closed to me. I had the very strong feeling that in order to take her hand I would have to start by seizing her arm and working my way downward to it, inch by inch. It had been making me feel uncertain and off-balance, as if her IQ was saying *hi there, big boy!* and her shoulders were saying *back off, buster.*

But I didn't see this so clearly at the time. I was just feeling hopeful and confused: give it time, I told myself. What I *was* aware of, though, was extraordinarily strange. *I could not figure out what she looked like.* I could not form a clear picture of her face in my mind. I was not sure how tall she was, or what color her hair was, or what her figure looked like, which was doubly strange because she wore wonderfully formfitting jeans and elegant jackets. Each time she came to her door it was as if I was seeing her for the first time.

It baffled me. How could I see someone several times and still have no idea what she looked like? Her online photo was no help because it didn't look like her *at all.* It looked like a bad waxwork sculpture of her. Even the *camera* couldn't capture her.

There was a definite sense of energy on our fourth date that hadn't been there before. However, there was one hitch. I'd sprained my vocal cords from having shouted too loudly at a party a few weeks before, and I'd been sucking down cough drops for days. I'd taken a few during our conversation, and as I drove her home I grew uncertain. By now my mouth was an air-conditioner blast of mentho-lyptus. If I grossed her out, it could be the end. So I decided to play it safe. There was no rush, I figured. In the car, I leaned over to kiss her cheek. At the very last instant she turned her face full toward me, there was a flurry and a confusion, and it dawned on me one millisecond too late that she *would* have kissed me.

Driving home, I felt both very stupid and very thrilled. "She *would* have kissed me," I said to myself, grinning. "She *would* have."

But in the comedy of dating, so much gets decided in an instant. It's like figure skating, where the smallest error, the slightest misstep, can destroy all the effort that has gone before. She *gave* me permission at last, and I seemingly turned it down. On our fifth date, she smiled but her attention seemed elsewhere. She spoke of wondering if she could afford to stay in San Francisco, which made my heart sink. At her door I *did* kiss her this time, but it was a dry kiss, no energy in it, no passion.

Things came to a head on our sixth date. I took her to an expensive restaurant in Palo Alto. She was more cautious and guarded than ever, and sensing that, I was exaggeratedly attentive and polite. It was all out of whack. I took her back to my apartment and poured some wine and set out some chocolate. Finally, resignedly, I put things out in the open. "I'd really like to kiss you," I said, "but I just don't know where we stand."

At that point she was perched on the far end of my couch, legs clamped together, shoulders hunched, staring down at her hands with a stricken look on her face. All of a sudden, I felt like I was torturing Bambi.

"I just don't feel the chemistry," she said in a small voice, not meeting my eyes.

"Oh," I said. I groaned and slumped sideways on the couch. When a woman says that, a man is finished. It's the Black Death of dating. There's no recovery from a line like that.

A few moments went by in silence. *O God,* I thought to myself, *I did everything I could, she's so marvelous, and I'm still going to lose.*

"Do you want me to leave?" she said, still addressing her hands, her face even paler than usual.

I might have gotten angry then, the way I did with Sharon. I might have tried to make her feel guilty. But as I learned from Sharon, love is like grace. It's not something you can demand or even earn. For some men it may be a survival trait to pressure women to get what they want. But I am part-animal, part-computer now, genus unknown, and perhaps I am so new that the species just doesn't know what to do with me. My body is so strange, even to myself, that I just do not know what the universe thinks my survival value is. And so my only rational choice was to be willing to lose with honor, because then someday I could also win with honor.

Gently, I said, "No, Laura, I don't want you to leave." The entire sentence was a sustained sigh. I got up and went to the kitchen to give her some space and breathing room. I brought her back some water, because it seemed like the right thing to do.

To defuse the mood I told her the story of my very first rejection, in seventh grade. We were in a summer enrichment class. After several weeks of furtive adoration I had finally managed to catch her alone after class. In an unsteady, quavering voice, I had said something like, "Uh . . . after class sometime, would you like to go for a sandwich?" So much blood had drained out of my face that the fluorescent lights overhead seemed unnaturally bright. She had gasped, clapped both hands to her mouth, turned around, and run away down the hall either screaming, or laughing, or both. The fire doors had *flupped* shut behind her. I was left all alone, doing my best not to pass out.

"What else could I do?" I said to Laura, twenty-five years later. "I walked all the way home, crawled under my bedcovers, and stayed there till morning."

The story wasn't done, though, until I told her the capper. "The next day, she spent the entire class session furiously scribbling insulting notes and passing them to me. The one I remember was an outline of a head with a small dot scribbled inside it, and she'd written above it, 'Your brain is *this big*.'"

While I was telling this story, Laura's body language had changed. She'd turned to face me, drawing both knees up onto the couch. Smiling.

"And you know what?" I said. "What I didn't know at that age is that *any* attention from a twelve-year-old girl equals flirting. I totally missed the underlying message. She *was* interested."

Laura laughed.

"I could have bagged her," I said, shaking my head. "Could've done it. At thirteen. And my entire adult life would have been different."

I walked her out to her car. She gave me a hug. "Write me soon," she said.

We got together for a hike in a Silicon Valley park several weeks later, so that we could talk without the overhanging dread of it being a date. A no-bullshit conversation; a postmortem.

A light drizzle began to fall as she tried to explain why she had been so ambivalent. The vast hillside between us and the sea was draped in a moody beauty, bunched up in more versions of green than my eye had channels to count. Soon the weather went from drizzle to rain, and our shoes began to squelch in mud. My umbrella wouldn't open and I fussed with it in growing confusion, unable to figure out what little latch or catch had gone awry. Finally I gave up. "*You* hold it a second," I said, shrugging off my knapsack so I could pack it away. When she took it, it blossomed open instantly. We stared at each other incredulously, then began laughing. It was the Divine Feminine at work. Normally it maketh the fallow field to bloom, but sometimes it also fixeth the occasional household appliance.

That day, she told me of sorrows in her past that helped me understand why she sometimes walked with her shoulders protectively hunched inward, and why she was so acutely able to differentiate between looks that were predatory or appreciative. She could not avoid being stared at on the street, but she could make herself invisible to a man's inner eye. I will always remember her face and the angle of her hips as she sat on my couch, smiling at me as I told the story of one of the great humiliations of my teenage life. It's just a little sliver of vision, though, like glimpsing her for an instant through a door cracked open an inch. She told me she's a "strawberry blonde," but I can't see in my mind what color her hair is. I still have no idea, at all, what color her eyes are.

The computer had brought us together. The computer had no parameters that could quantify *zing*. When a man and a woman face each other across the table for the first time they have nothing but data to buttress them. No shared memories from which a decades-long conversation can take root, nothing from which the courage to take a hand can be kindled. There is only the strained jockeying for position, peering through the brittle mask of the Other. Hothousing love by pumping data into it. I was informed by one redheaded beauty that I was the *sixty-eighth* man she had dated that year. "Dating is a numbers game," she told me, primly. "I hope I'm better than number sixty-seven," I wisecracked to hide my astonishment. The tyranny of choice really *is* tyranny. I might blame my frustrations on being short and deaf were it not that men of brawny shoulders and women of slender grace seem to have little better luck, in the end, than I do. They may bed more often, but they always seem to break up six months later. Love is fragile and easily broken without the grounding soil of clans and kinships and communities. They let people discover one another gradually over months and years in a slow and unhurried building of admiration and desire.

After that conversation with Laura, I began letting most of my online dating memberships expire. Bye, eHarmony and your psychological proctoscopies. Bye, match.com and your coiffed marketing bunnies, who all say they live for taking long walks on the beach. Bye, jdate, I've always done better with the shiksas anyway. But I kept my Salon Personals membership. Its members were smart and funny and literate. I might yet find that love is strong enough to take root even in the arid ground of ones and zeros.

But on the whole, the ascendancy of online dating and speed-dating is a sure sign that our society has surrendered its soul to the logic of *if-then-else*. That logic has spread its tendrils into every aspect of daily life. It has suffocated and chilled the lives of many communities, and is set to destroy others outright. The signing deaf community is but one of the more obvious casualties. The prospect of conquering deafness with binary logic tears my heart with joy and grief in bewilderingly equal measure. Nineteenth-century Americans celebrated the dismembering of Indian tribes with thoughtless cheer. *Manifest Destiny*, they called it. Today we see it as tragedy. When twenty-second-century historians write the history of cochlear implants and the end of ASL, they may come to the same conclusion. However, they will not find malice. Not deliberate genocide. Only thousands of separately made rational decisions gradually accumulating into a computational tidal wave so overwhelming that even the clearest-eyed observers could only stand by in helpless wonder and sorrow.

9. A Kinship with the Machines

DANGER

STRONG MAGNETIC FIELD

NO METALLIC IMPLANTS

Persons with pacemakers, neurostimulators, or metallic implants must not enter the landscaped area. Serious injury may result.

— Sign in the flower garden above Stanford Hospital's MRI scanner

I HAD ACCEPTED the fact of exile. I had given up on the world ever sounding right again. But I wasn't *happy* about it.

A few days after I upgraded to Hi-Res, Vivian had put a teapot on the stove to boil, and after a while I started hearing a hoarse thrumming sound, like a foghorn.

"What *is* that?" I was watching the steam billow out, so it was a ridiculous question. But I was expecting a whistle, which was what I had heard with hearing aids, and this wasn't a whistle. Perhaps it was another loud sound that was happening at exactly the same time.

"It's the teapot," Vivian said, briskly turning it off.

I stared at it. "It sounded like a foghorn."

"Well, it's the teapot."

I said, "What does it sound like to you?"

"It sounds like a whistle."

Well, now it sounded like a foghorn. As the Chinese proverb says, a man with one watch knows the time, a man with two is never sure. Given multiple versions of auditory reality, how could I know which was the most real? A cyborg could be forgiven a certain degree of solipsism.

Actually, I did have *some* sense of the real. Certain sounds were so bizarre that I simply couldn't believe the processor was representing them accurately. On SAS, the microwave no longer had the high-pitched, monochromatic *beep beeep beeeeep* sound I'd heard all my life with hearing aids. It sounded like *braat braat braaaaaat.* If microwaves had babies this is what the infants would sound like, emitting static when they cried. Since other *beeps,* like those of telephones, sounded reasonably normal, I could only guess that the microwave was an aberration, a pitch whose frequency just happened to exploit a specific weakness of the processor's software. Later, I found that I was exactly right. When I upgraded to Hi-Res, the microwave suddenly sounded like *beeeeep* again, a pure clear tone. I asked one of the scientists about it and he said, "Yes. You were getting an aliasing effect." In other words, the microwave's frequency was close to an exact multiple of how often SAS refreshed the electrode array, throwing off the system's ability to represent it for the same reason that car tires in films appear to be going backward. SAS haplessly reproduced the sound "backward," giving me a completely wrong representation of it. Hi-Res's faster refresh rate made the aliasing effect go away.

But to a little kid growing up on SAS — and hundreds if not thousands of little kids have — *braaaaat* will *be* the microwave's sound. When they upgrade to newer software they may spend the rest of their lives feeling vaguely puzzled because the microwave never sounds right again.

Take, for another example, the *automatic gain control* — the part of my software that I talked about earlier. It boosts soft sounds and damps loud ones, but it is all too obviously a crude approximation of the way a normal ear does the same thing. It makes the hiss of the air-conditioning go away whenever I talk, and then when I stop, a third of a second elapses before *whoosh,* it comes back. For months I thought it was simply a focusing effect of my own mind, like the beat or two it takes for one's eyes to focus on a page of text. But Tony Spahr, a researcher at Arizona State, explained to me that no, it was my automatic gain control. When it's quiet, the AGC cranks up the microphone's sensitivity to pull in soft sounds. When a loud sound comes along, the software assumes it's important and decreases the sensitivity so that background noise doesn't wash it out. When the loud sound ceases for more than a third of a second, it cranks the sensitivity up again on the optimistic assumption that it's gone away for good.

It's touching: my software is following me around like an eager butler, constantly trying to help me out by tinkering with my settings. And I can *hear* it doing it. I have no objection to the logic, but it does have a certain deep-rooted effect on my perception of the world. Sounds I know to be continuous go away, then come back after an embarrassed little hiccup of silence.

Becoming a cyborg infects one with a certain rueful irony, because it overturns the blithe assumption that one's sensory organs deliver a truthful representation of the universe. They don't; one's most basic relationships to reality can be amended and edited and upgraded; reality is ultimately a matter of software. People with normal ears are not off the epistemological hook, because their "software" was written haphazard by millions of years of evolution and has no greater claim to reality. One can innocently believe in the real only with senses that are hard-wired and not easily changed. I know this fact up close and personal now, and the price I pay for it is that I have to stay out of the Garden.

"The cyborg would not recognize the Garden of Eden; it is not made of mud and cannot dream of returning to dust," Donna Haraway wrote in a much-read essay on the idea of the cyborg in 1985.* I first encountered the essay while taking a graduate seminar at Duke on postmodern cultural theory, and it had both captivated

* The interested reader may find this essay, "A Cyborg Manifesto," on the Web.

and mystified me. The sheer wistfulness of that statement about Eden had resonated deeply with me, although I could barely understand what it meant. I thought of Eden as that place where perception revealed the truth about reality, where one could speak the language that gave everything its true name. From that Eden, I was now in exile. The fields of my ears had been destroyed. I had stumbled in a field of tall grass, and fallen. Polysyllabic little signs now ringed the garden, saying DANGER.

But Haraway's essay fascinated me because it seemed to say, in its sheer opaque poetry, that there was something *good* about being a cyborg, about being cast out of Eden. It was not the false absolution of emotional rigidity, the choice Joey had made in becoming a robot. It was not the alienation and violence of the so-called cyborg in *The Terminator*. Wrote Haraway, "Cyborg imagery can suggest a way out of the maze of dualisms in which we have explained our bodies and our tools to ourselves." I liked the idea of finding my way out of "mazes of dualisms." But the essay had resisted my efforts to understand it. What was I to make of Delphic pronouncements like this? . . .

> The cyborg is a creature in a post-gender world; it has no truck with bisexuality, pre-oedipal symbiosis, unalienated labour, or other seductions to organic wholeness through a final appropriation of all the powers of the parts into a higher unity. In a sense, the cyborg has no origin story in the Western sense — a "final" irony since the cyborg is also the awful apocalyptic telos of the "West's" escalating dominations of abstract individuation, an ultimate self untied at last from all dependency, a man in space.

Let me get this straight — Steve Austin was supposed to have "no truck with pre-oedipal symbiosis"? I reread the essay shortly after activation but found myself unable to decide, once again, whether it was postmodernist bullshit, socialist rant, manic Nietzschean poetry, sly parody, brilliant cultural theory, or (quite possibly) all of the above. Haraway's characterization of the cyborg seemed alien to my experience. After all, with the singular exception of my implant, I was very definitely made of mud and had often dreamed, fearfully, of returning to dust; I was by no means untied from all dependency, indeed precisely the opposite was true; and if I could be the awful apocalyptic telos of *anything*, I hoped somebody would let me know. It sounded like fun.

My feelings about the essay ran deeper than just confusion. I felt resentment as well. I had been exiled from Duke because I had not been able to talk or write like this. In the early 1990s, its graduate English department had become the top department in the country for literary theory. I had somehow gotten in, but had never felt at home.* I had struggled mightily to understand various theorists and theories, including deconstruction, reader-response, New Historicism, and postmodernism. I'd gotten good grades and even scored a couple of conference papers and publications, but I had always felt like a dog trying to speak cat. I knew that literary theorists were trying to use language to explore the limitations of language, a staggeringly difficult task, and much of their seeming opacity came from pushing language to its limits to see where it broke down. The collective enterprise was as profound, in its own way, as metamathematics or quantum mechanics. But all I could do was sit on the sidelines and watch the game, gleaning some of its pleasure secondhand, instead of actually playing it. My own writing remained stubbornly untheoretical and jargon-free. When I did try to use jargon, my words felt clumsy and amateurish, like I was trying to do surgery with mittens.

Things came to a head in 1993 at my "preliminary examination," an oral exam to see how well I understood various works and theories. Passing the exam was a prerequisite for beginning my dissertation. I can barely remember what happened during the two hours or so it lasted. The one question I remember being asked is, "What is representation?" (It might have been Stanley Fish who asked

* By the way, I was entirely unaware that at the same time Blake Wilson, Michael Pierschalla, and their colleagues were hard at work developing CIS not three hundred yards away from the English department's building.

that one.) I was utterly unable to answer. I failed the exam, spectacularly. It melted down my academic career, and for a long time, my self-respect. Shattered and humiliated, I had dropped out of the program.

And so Haraway's essay felt like a letter written directly to me (I was an actual cyborg now, for goodness' sake), but in a language I had failed to learn. I found myself rebelling, once again, at the density of its jargon, its uncompromising difficulty. But I also felt that Haraway was saying something important that I *had* to understand in order to learn to live in a body whose senses had to be evaluated by their usefulness rather than by their fidelity to the material world. Through 2002 and 2003 I reread it again, and again, and again.

I slowly realized that for Haraway, the story of the Garden of Eden is crucial for understanding the cyborg. References to the Garden and the Fall permeate the essay. The story of Eden is a lie, Haraway says, because there never *was* an Eden. She writes, "But with the loss of innocence in our origin, there is no expulsion from the Garden either . . . Cyborg writing must not be about the Fall, the imagination of a once-upon-a-time wholeness before language, before writing, before Man." Haraway was saying the same thing as David Hume: humans have never had an original wholeness, never had a true perception of reality. Modern neurobiology fully backs them up on this point (and Haraway is, by the way, a biologist by training). We saw earlier that when soft sounds are detected by the inner hair cells, the outer hair cells feed fresh energy into the system to amplify the neural reaction to the sound. On the other end of the auditory scale, when an extremely loud sound hits the eardrum a small muscle called the *stapedius* automatically contracts, stiffening the eardrum to damp it. That is why the decibel scale is logarithmic, because sounds that are in fact thousands of times louder than others seem, to human ears, only a few score times as loud. (Incidentally, the same is true of vision as well.) Hume would have been delighted to learn of it. Dear reader with organic ears, *you do not perceive the world the way it actually is, and you never will.* But be glad: a truly faithful rendition of the auditory world would either be flat and shallow, or unbearably painful.

I had learned, viscerally, how constructed my perception was. My body's "original language" had been shattered into a post-Babelian heterogeneity of codes. Experiencing the world through CIS, SAS, and Hi-Res had destroyed my innocent belief that the senses gave a veridical representation of the world. As Haraway says, the cyborg is forced by its own body into permanent skepticism about the perception of reality.

Which makes the cyborg a figure of hope, Haraway argues, because it is inherently immune to the lie of Eden. Viewing the universe from multiple perspectives makes it more able to resist ideologies that claim that their way of viewing reality is the only one. Cyborgs are even more fallen than most. But that is cause for hope rather than despair, because giving up the search for the Garden liberates us to build *gardens* — no-caps, plural.

That's all very theoretical, even if you buy it: okay, multiple perspectives are better. How, exactly, could I use that knowledge to build gardens — that is, a world I could be happy with despite its incompleteness? My new body gave me a clue. Haraway's cultural theory also works on a purely perceptual level. Most people with cochlear implants, including me, have them in only one ear, leaving the other ear deaf. Being one-eared is really very practical. With half the cost, half the surgical risk, and half the batteries you get about 80 percent of the benefit of two ears. (Think how much you could still do in life with only one eye.) Why bother, then, to implant both ears, as a few people have done in clinical trials? It's not easy to justify in financial terms, and the FDA and the insurance companies are still pondering whether to make it standard practice. But an audiologist working on clinical trials at one of the implant companies told me that their bilateral patients greatly appreciated having two ears instead of one. When I asked why, she paused, unable to trot out a thoroughly validated scientific rationale. "They feel more *connected* to the world," she said, and paused again to think it over some more. "They say they feel more *alive.* They just *love* it." I could tell from her face that she wasn't just feeding me a company line (a fair concern, given that profits from bilateral implantation are, of course, doubled). These were real people she was talking about, people whom she had come to know well. Connection, joy, pleasure, a sense of being richly part of the world — these are not measurable in a testing booth, which gives the FDA fits.

And yet they are as real as any scientific data one can muster. A man with one watch knows the time; a man with two is never sure. But the man with two has a more interesting life. He knows that human knowledge is contingent and constructed, always provisional and open to renegotiation. Having binaural hearing lets you know, in the most visceral terms, the freedom that comes from having multiple perspectives on reality. I know that as a one-eared person, I'm missing that richness. But the process of having gone through different kinds of software has re-created that perspective to some extent. It's let me triangulate on reality the same way a one-eyed man can produce an approximation of depth perception by moving his head from side to side. As a cyborg with a programmable ear I have acquired new senses of freedom, both auditory and political. Hi-Res sounds no more "real" to me than SAS, but my test scores suggest that I am finding it more *useful.* On SAS, I could identify 17 percent of the words in sentences spoken against a stiff background of white noise. In February 2003, on Hi-Res, my score was 39 percent. An upgrade, indeed.

I was beginning to agree with Haraway that the story of Eden was a lie, and a lie with consequences, most of them bad. Trying to get back into Eden was not just misguided; it was disastrous. Politicians gain power by claiming that they offer the One True Way to know the world. To the masses they offer certitude, resolve, power. But it is only the appearance of power. A perspective that sorts everything in the world into good and evil is itself the greatest possible evil because it blinds the storyteller to the complexity and multidimensionality of the world. The bits and pieces of academic jargon Haraway uses — "pre-oedipal symbiosis, unalienated labour," and so forth — all refer caustically to *master narratives*, that is, various theories of a single unitary Truth through which all reality can be described. "Single vision produces worse illusions than double vision or many-headed monsters," Haraway writes.

An immense amount of destruction has been caused by people with single vision and master narratives. Examples abound, but I will speak here only of deafness. Harlan Lane's insistence that sign language is the only valid alternative for deaf children was a classic single-vision stance, demonizing the medical community, as was the Council of Milan's decree in 1880 that all deaf children should be educated orally, casting the speakers of ASL beyond the pale. Both stances have had catastrophic consequences for generations of real, live children.

To have single vision is to be a monster. Hollywood knows this in an extraordinarily literal sense. Virtually all of its evil robots and cyborgs have but one eye. When the Terminator is wounded, the viewer's gaze is drawn to its hideously exposed robotic eye — it is now revealed as a moral Cyclops. *Star Trek*'s totalitarian Borg villains always have one eye concealed, plugged into some sort of data feed. Robocop, whose helmet combines his eyes into a single slit, is touted as the ultimate police officer because he has the entire corpus of the law in his memory banks. As if simply having the rulebook enabled one to make perfect decisions! Robocop might dispense justice but not mercy, and therefore, in the end, no justice. Robocop becomes a sympathetic character only when he sheds his helmet, enabling the viewer to see both of his (human) eyes. The hybridity of the cyborg, its profane fusion of the human and the mechanical, symbolizes a politics that does not try to impose a single unidimensional view of Truth on the world. The one intolerable perspective is the belief that there is only *one* perspective. The National Association for the Deaf's new position statement in 2000 recognizing the validity of cochlear implantation is literally a cyborg politics, in its acceptance of human-machine fusions and linguistic diversity.

Time to abandon Eden, then. Master narratives are human constructions of a reality that has no human dimension. The universe has neither masters nor narratives. It simply *is.* Even science, that supposed paragon of objectivity and truth, is a human construction of reality. The division of the ear's neurology into place, rate, and phase coding is an analytical convenience rather than a veridical model of the way the ear works. The auditory system is so incredibly complicated and recursive that we have to settle for partial constructs of it to make any progress at all. From the listener's perspective, the ear doesn't have three coding schemas — it has *one.* (You don't feel as if you hear three versions of the world simultaneously, do you?) To scientists, science doesn't feel like flooding a dark cave with light; it feels like exploring it with a single candle, seeing little bits of it at a time. And the hell of it is, there are no arrows on the floor showing you where you should look next. Depending on your interests, you can go *this* way or *that* way, and if you go *that* way, you will never find out what you might have discovered had you gone *this* way. Whichever way you choose, you will leave huge areas of the cave forever unexplored and unlit. The experience is humbling, excruciating, terrifying. In my dissertation research, there was a point where I came to the appalling realization that something as trivial as the order in which I read papers was having a profound impact on how I was organizing my chapters and building code. Paper A changed the way I read paper B; if I'd read paper B first, I would have read A differently or decided not to read A at all, and the dissertation would have gone in a different direction as a result. The number of possible dissertations I could write was beyond computation. I would end up writing *one* of them. Just *one.*

Faced with that kind of crisis, one has at least three alternatives. One can go mad (some do: in 1889 Nietzsche was found sobbing on a horse's neck, and spent the remainder of his life officially insane). One can withdraw from the search for knowledge into the false safety of dogma. Or one can choose to see the multivalence of the universe as an invitation to explore and play. The latter choice makes one ironic but not cynical, because play is always an expression of hope. One can choose to work with what is revealed by one's candle. To do so is to take responsibility for one's choices between *this* and *that.* To live sanely in a cyborg body, one has to learn how to make choices. Haraway writes,

> A cyborg body is not innocent; it was not born in a garden; it does not seek unitary identity and so generate antagonistic dualisms without end (or until the world ends); it takes irony for granted . . . The machine is not an it to be animated, worshipped, and dominated. The machine is us, our processes, an aspect of our embodiment. We can be responsible for machines; they do not dominate or threaten us.

By now I had learned to give up my quest for a unitary identity. In speaking of the cyborg as "an ultimate self untied at last from all dependency," that is precisely what Haraway is resisting rather than holding up for approval. In place of *The Terminator's* nightmare world, where cyborgs are confused with robots, she offers a positive vision of cyborgs as profoundly *human,* profoundly connected to the world:

> From another perspective, a cyborg world might be about lived social and bodily realities in which people are not afraid of their joint kinship with animals and machines, not afraid of permanently partial identities and contradictory standpoints.

Haraway's essay now struck me as a straightforward description of my life. I experienced joint kinship with animals and machines, feeling oddly affectionate toward my robot vacuum cleaner yet also reveling in the smells and lusts of my animal body. I was permanently and pleasurably adrift in eternal uncertainty about teapots and microwaves. Cyborgs "have no truck" with master narratives because there is no single story running their bodies. My sensory universe is now constructed by squadrons of programmers, not the garden fields of my ear. Unitary identity? Not anymore, if ever;

there are two minds in my skull, one built by my genes, the other by a corporation. I am a walking collective, a community of at least two. The x-rays of my head are riveting, a stark juxtaposition of sensuous biology and angular computational power. The computer invaded the sacred domain of my body, yet to my own astonishment we learned to work together as a total system, mutually changing each other in the process. I fed it lithium-ion batteries; it fed me electrons. I altered its software; it repatterned the dendrites in my auditory cortex. We have *literally* reprogrammed each other. And while I *am* made of mud, my implant's ceramic casing will not return to dust. If my grave is exhumed by curious anthropologists twenty thousand years from now, it may be the only part of me that is left.

It was not that I had acquired a postmodern way of thinking. It was that I had acquired a postmodern *body.* It had taught me what I could not grasp when I was at Duke. To the question "What is representation?" I would now answer, "Representation is the act of creating an interpretation of an otherwise unknowable reality." I couldn't have said that in 1993 because deep down, I wouldn't have believed it — and so I had quite rightly failed the test. Had the committee charitably passed me, I would have gone on to write a mediocre dissertation trying miserably to read Shakespeare through the lens of postmodern theories of language. I would never have gotten an academic job.

After that failure — that Fall — I spent the next year teaching computer courses. At a conference I ran into a friend who told me about a new program at the University of Texas at Austin where computers were being used to teach courses in English literature. Computers and literature: perfect. I applied, got in, and moved to Austin. When I was finishing up my dissertation in 1999 I was hired by a dot-com at probably twice the salary I would have commanded as an assistant professor.

While Martin Caidin's *Cyborg* gave me a model for how to *become* a cyborg, Haraway's "Manifesto" gave me a model for how to *be* a cyborg. In 1959, a schizophrenic Joey pretended to plug himself into electrical outlets and various gadgets to keep his body running. In 2003, I was doing that for real. But the psychological experience was completely different from what Joey had imagined, for he had chosen to be a robot, not a cyborg. My bionic hearing made me neither omniscient nor dehumanized: it made me more human, because I was constantly aware that my perception of the universe was provisional, the result of human decisions that would be revised time and again. Unlike Robocop or the Borg I was not disconnected from the world, remote and uncaring in the bioelectronic shell of my skin. The very provisionality of my perception reminded me that my political perspective was provisional also, and that it was my task as a human being to strive to connect ever more complexly and deeply with the people and places of my life.

Sunday. It was a beautiful mid-summer afternoon in 2003, and I was out in the backyard shoring up the tomatoes with stakes. Every cyborg should have a garden. Having a garden teaches you that living things have their own ideas about how to grow and develop, and the best one can do is provide support where it seems to be needed. I used thumbtacks for pegging string to the stakes, but then I ran out: I needed just one more. I rummaged in my drawer and smiled as I found a tie clip I bought ages ago, made out of a Pentium III microprocessor sold as jewelry in the gift shop at Intel's headquarters in Santa Clara. It would make a perfect thumbtack. In the dimming cool of the day, I pushed it into the soft wood of a stake and wrapped string around it to support the last tomato plant. The tomatoes hung heavy and red and low. The chip glittered in the last rays of the sun, a complicated little square of gold. My cyborg garden.

10. A Kinship with the Humans

It is not hearing that one misses but overhearing.

— DAVID WRIGHT, *Deafness*

IN MY WRITING GROUP, Joe Quirk was writing a novel about hang-gliding. It wasn't just a sport, but an encounter with the Divine. "I turn rainforests into chopsticks," his protagonist proclaimed while in flight. "I burrow deepest, race fastest, fly highest, flourish in every climate, exploit mysterious tradings of electrons. I have ascended heaven, and Eden is my toilet."

I was hooked, but months went by before I began to know Joe as a person. It started in 2003 when a mutual friend, Cheyenne, invited us both to go hiking in Palo Alto. The conversation turned to the important subject of how difficult it is to find a really good submarine sandwich in Silicon Valley, and I lamented being so far from the best sandwich shop in the universe, which is back where I grew up in New Jersey.

"Where in New Jersey?" Joe said suddenly.

"Westfield," I said.

"*Westfield!?*"

"Uh, yeah," I said warily. The name "Westfield" and a tone of astonishment don't usually go together.

"*I* grew up in Westfield!"

"Westfield High School?" I said.

"Yeah! 1984!"

"Huh," I said. "1983."

A bit of high-speed data exchange followed, which was gibberish to poor Cheyenne.

"Quagliano?"

"No, what about Aers?"

"Roy?"

"Not her, what about Keane?"

"Kevin Keane? The English teacher?"

"Yeah," he said. "Changed my whole life. I became an English major because of him. Made me want to be a writer."

"Me too," I said. It was so strange to hear his name coming out of Joe's mouth. "Keane was amazing. Incredibly cynical man. Brilliant teacher."

We stared at one another.

"How come we never knew each other?" I said. I had been co-editor of the school paper. I wasn't invited to many parties, but at least I knew all the names. And "Joe Quirk" is not a name one forgets readily.

"Oh," he said, "I was a Project 79 fuck-up."

"*You?* But . . . but . . . you're brilliant. How could you be in the remedial program?"

"Like I said, I was a fuck-up."

The best friendships develop slowly, with a sense of surprise and mystery. It took several more months for me to understand how a writer with Joe's talent could have been a Project 79 fuck-up. I slowly pieced it together as we began going out for burritos after the writing group. It wasn't a happy story: difficult childhood, lack of support and encouragement, and just plain being differently wired. But his first novel, *The Ultimate Rush*, was a pyrotechnic delight to read. I also went through his manuscript on sociobiology, *From Monkey Business to Marriage*, and found that not only was it rigorously researched but also maniacally funny and philosophically deep. He compared a spermatozoa meeting the egg to "a submarine crashing into San Francisco to deliver a pizza." The simile made me laugh aloud in delight, but there was also a distinctive philosophical sensibility running through the book. *Nature doesn't give a shit about our hopes and dreams,* his book said, *but our biological heritage makes it evolutionarily advantageous for us to have those hopes and dreams anyway.* We become human both because of and despite nature — a painful paradox.

As I got to know Joe, a tightly wound cord in my soul began to loosen. A year before, I would have defined a friendship with a man as wasted time. Of course I had close male friends elsewhere in the country, guys I'd known for a quarter-century, but making new male friends was at the bottom of my priority list. But Joe and I turned out to be spiritual twins. We are both differently wired, *Quirky* to use Joe's word, shaped by the crevices of confining childhoods, both curiously competent and bumbling at the same time. The synchrony of our lives was eerie. Not only did we have the same English teacher who had the same impact on both of us, we'd also gone to college in the same city, Providence, and ended up in California. He'd graduated in the bottom 10 percent of his class at Providence College. Then he'd read every book extant on sociobiology and wrote a brilliant and uniquely personal synthesis of it. He didn't fuck up. It was the educational system that had fucked up.

The gift unasked for, unmerited: the gift Michael Pierschalla gave to me before he died. He made furniture, and he helped make me. I have a mother and father, but I would also say that I now have *fabers.* The word *faber* in Latin means "craftsman" or "artisan." I felt a moral obligation to be a test subject myself, to pass on the gift that my *fabers* gave to me.

In the summer of 2004 I went down to Advanced Bionics to let Jerry Loeb and Leo Litvak try out their theories on me. Jerry Loeb used to be the chief scientist at Advanced Bionics, which most definitely made him one of my *fabers.* He looked exactly like what you would get if you took an eager sixteen-year-old Jewish kid out of a science fair in the Bronx and added a dusting of gray to his curly hair in a futile attempt to age him up a bit. He'd sent me one of his articles several months before, dated 1983, and had written across the top, "This is where the Clarion started." ("Clarion" is the brand name of my implant.) Leafing through it, I saw what he meant: it was an engineering blueprint, full of diagrams and polysyllabic words such as *anisotropic, parylene, methacrylate,* and *silastic.* Much of the design was well out of date, but that only reinforced how pioneering the paper was. The implant embedded in my body evolved over decades of trial and error, arguments, controversies, and — yes — mistakes. If they had been afraid to make mistakes, there would *be* no implant.

On the evening of our appointment, Jerry had driven up from USC, where he now worked, to join forces with Leo Litvak, an engineer at Advanced Bionics. If Jerry was the old hand, the experienced pioneer, then Leo was the bright young newcomer — although, to look at them, one could be forgiven for thinking it was the other way around. Leo's demeanor was gentle, shy, and inward, and he moved tentatively, as if slightly embarrassed to be caught living in the material world of computers and oscilloscopes. He wore the dark pants, white shirt, and yarmulke of an Orthodox Jew, so that if someone had shown me a picture of him and told me that it had been taken in 1902, I would have believed it. But I had read his dissertation on cochlear implant programming, which he completed at MIT in 2002, and his writing was so bold and clear and lucid that it was obvious why Advanced Bionics had hired him instantly. Leo was a rising star with the shy smile of a gentle devotee.

So there we were, three Jews of various flavors, concocting scientific incantations in northern L.A. We'd commandeered a conference room and spread out Leo's laptop, Jerry's synthesizer piano keyboard, various bits of expensive handmade electronic equipment, and since it was past dinnertime, a half green-pepper, half black-olive pizza.

Their goal, Jerry told me, was to get around one of the key barriers to writing better software: the implant's inability to reproduce phase coding. In phase coding, hair cells fire "in phase" with sound waves sweeping up the cochlea. But in my ear, there were no hair cells to be triggered. The electrode array had nothing to sweep.

That meant there was no way to replicate the normal ear's wave motion. The best the implant could do was replace the "wind" bending the hair cells with strong puffs of "air" (that is, electricity) beamed straight down at the nerve endings. The result was a signal that users' brains found confusingly static, because the brain has evolved to handle the "sweep" of hair cells firing in sequence as sound waves travel up the cochlea. Jerry and Leo couldn't replicate the wave motion, but they thought they could at least break up the static character of the signal with high pulse rates in order to evoke more lifelike nerve activity. So today they were going to stimulate my cochlea at high pulse rates to see what would happen.

"Uh, what sort of pulse rates are we talking about here?" I asked a little nervously as Leo plugged my processor into his laptop. The software I was running was Hi-Res, which had a pulse rate of 5,156 times per second.

"Up to about twenty thousand pulses per second," Leo said absently. He was staring intensely into his screen. Moving around sliders, pulling down menus, tapping in numbers. Getting ready to reboot me.

"A pulse rate that high won't electrocute me, right?"

"No, the voltage's the same, it's only the pulse rate that's different."

Twenty thousand pulses per second into my tender little cochlea. Okay . . . okay . . .

"And what's *that* going to sound like?" I asked. Just sort of, generally, in round terms, you know.

Leo beamed at me gently. "That's what we need you to tell us."

Oh. Right.

While Leo continued setting up, Jerry explained some more. "We know you'll hear beeps. What we want to know is what the beeps sound like to you. We'll play them in pairs, and we'll ask you which of the two sounds louder, or more high-pitched. We'll also ask you to tell us which key on the piano sounds closest to some of the pitches you hear."

"Okay," I said, reaching for a slice of pizza. If I was about to be exposed to twenty thousand pulses per second, I needed to do a little carbo-loading first. "I can do that."

When Leo asked, "Ready?" I nodded. Then all of a sudden, I was in silence. Leo had just overridden my software. He was now running my ear out of his laptop. He did something with his keyboard. I heard:

beep *beep*

"Sound 2 is higher-pitched," I said.

And we were off and running. Many, many pairs of beeps followed. Then I carefully compared various beeps against keys on the piano, zeroing in as best I could on the closest matches. My responses would let Jerry and Leo correlate between patterns of stimulation and my perceptual experience. I felt a great sense of responsibility to get it right, because their theories could only be as good as the data that informed them. Bad data would lead to bad theories. I often asked Leo to play a given *beep* several times so that I could confirm that my best guess really *was* my best guess.

Frequently Leo turned me back on (that is, restored my normal software) so that we could all discuss what they wanted me to listen for. Most of Jerry and Leo's back-and-forth conversation during these times was so technical that I had only the vaguest idea what they were talking about. When Leo overrode my software I had *no* idea, because then I couldn't hear anything but the *beeps* from his laptop. For long periods I just had to wait in silence while they hashed things out between themselves, deciding what to do next. Then I felt like a robot that had been switched off while its creators discussed its technical specs. I could see Leo's and Jerry's lips move, and I was aware that the air between them was full of sound energy and information, but it was a remote, dreamlike experience. I wasn't exactly a *thing* at such moments, but I was no longer a factor in the living human world, either. It was a familiar experience, because dozens of times in my life I have sat alone in soundproof booths while audiologists pore over the data produced by my responses, making calculations and decisions in what is, to me, utter silence.

It was more than a familiar experience. It was a familiar *feeling.* One of my earliest memories is of a dream in which I was sitting on the toilet with a pair of large, heavy headphones on my ears. I don't remember any of the hearing tests I had as a young child, much less my toilet training, but I remember the dreams I had about them later on. In this dream my mother and another woman were talking intensely between themselves, tête-à-tête, while rows of red lights blinked rhythmically on the wall behind them, as if we were all in a spaceship. They were discussing what to do with me. I was terrified that they were deciding whether to flush me away; I imagined my body folding up like a ruler and *flooshing* down the whirlpool. But all I could do was sit there, my feet heavy in Buster Brown suede shoes, awaiting my verdict in silence. I still feel a chilly residue of that dream every time I am in a soundproof booth or hooked up to a scientist's laptop. I am nearly forty now, but every time the years drop away and I am back in the mind of the frightened three-year-old animal I was in 1967.

Now Jerry and Leo wanted to know how the beeps sounded different from each other. I ransacked my word-hoard. After a while, I started to sound like a snooty wine taster. This one's got more depth than the other, I said. That one's got a sort of metallic edge. This one's got a more rarefied, distant quality. Jerry was writing all this down with a look on his face that said, *Well, maybe someday we'll understand what he means by all this.*

So far, so good, I figured. But then we got to a point where all the pairs sounded exactly the same, and I was saying "Identical" over and over again. By my fourth or fifth "Identical," Leo was cradling his chin in his hand, staring at his laptop computer with what could only be described as a dismayed poker face.

He looked over at Jerry. There was a long pause. I started to feel a little guilty.

"I gather this is not what you expected," I said cautiously.

Time out. Jerry gestured at Leo to turn my ear on, and in a moment I was back in the world of the human.

"It's not that you're messing up our theory, Mike," Jerry said kindly. "We don't really *have* a theory yet that you can mess up. So little is known about this kind of stimulation that almost any result can surprise us."

"Mmm," I said sympathetically, doing the only thing I could at the moment, which was to take another bite of pizza.

"Some of my smartest graduate students get freaked out when they discover what our lives are really like," Jerry went on. "They think science is about asking questions and devising experiments that answer them. They think there is a map to knowledge they can follow by just working hard. But the truth is that we often don't even know what the right *questions* are. There *is* no map. Some of my students get so disoriented by this that they have to quit and do something else."

But successful scientists are familiar with disorientation. To Jerry science was not a predictable march from ignorance to knowledge, but eternal play in the fields of data. I have found that the scientists I trust the most are the ones who have that enchanting combination of humility and playfulness. As Jerry explained, I realized that he and Leo were exploring at the limits of their own understanding. They were hoping that as they tried this kind of stimulation with more people, a pattern would emerge that would enable them to create a workable theory. "Then," Jerry told me with a glint of mad-scientist humor, "we'll be able to run experiments whose results will support that theory, and we'll publish a paper which will make it look like we thought of the theory first and then collected data that happened to prove it. But what you're seeing here today is the way it really works, Leo and I looking at each other in confusion and saying, 'What's going on here?'"

What was going on that evening, as the clock's big hand crept from five to six to seven to eight to nine P.M., was that Leo and Jerry and I were a team, each of us contributing our backgrounds and skills to the long effort of defeating a human scourge. That made me a *faber* as well, in a small but real way. Perhaps a few lines of the code that will be running inside the children at my old preschool for the deaf five or ten years from now will be different, and better, because of me. They may inherit a little bit of my mind, my software DNA.

Working with Jerry and Leo, I felt both the glory and the sorrow of being a cyborg. The glory came from living in so many fascinating new versions of reality, and working with brilliant people creating extraordinary devices. I was part of the work now.

The sorrow came from having been cut off from the living human world for all those years, and from being in a body that could be cut off even now. When I am switched off I revert to the mute little animal that still lives on in my dreams. That animal is as embedded in my spirit as the machine logic installed in my skull. I can never, ever escape it. I am part computer and part animal, and in ways that are both thrilling and lonely, the combination of the two makes me entirely human.

The next day, I was scheduled to give a talk at Advanced Bionics's quarterly research meeting. Van Harrison, the company's vice president of R&D, had asked me to speak about my experiences as an implant user. I'd said sure, expecting that I'd be sitting around a table with ten or twelve technical people.

But I found that the meeting was in the cafeteria. The *cafeteria?* When I got there people were streaming in from both ends of the room, taking up all the tables, standing up around the walls. They just kept coming. Soon there were, oh my God, at least 150 people in the room. Van's executive assistant was setting up trays of steaming chicken and garlic bread by the sink; other people were setting up a podium and sound system. Numbly I got in line for lunch, frantically organizing a whole new talk in my head. *Oh, shit, the acoustics are terrible.* Tiled floor, hard walls. What if I couldn't hear questions? And they'd built my ear. It was going to be so embarrassing.

But I wasn't on the firing line just yet. Several speakers came before me, and I listened with fascination because this was insider stuff. Completely new products, having nothing to do with hearing but drawing on their expertise in neurostimulation from developing cochlear implants, were in the pipeline. One speaker talked with tough-minded frankness about problems the company faced in growing. This was the Advanced Bionics I had come to know. Two years before, the company had gone through a traumatic period when several patients had contracted meningitis, a deadly disease, after implantation and died. Suspicion alighted on a particular component of the device, the *positioner*, a little plastic shim inserted behind the electrode array to push it closer to the nerves in the center of the cochlea. I had a positioner. Naturally, I was concerned. Shortly after the news came out I got a certified letter from the company explaining the issue and the risks in clear and precise terms and recommending that I get vaccinated for meningitis. For several months the company suspended selling the device entirely and then reintroduced it, minus positioner.

I got myself vaccinated, and then, because the numbers were small — out of tens of thousands of implant surgeries worldwide, ninety-one cases and seventeen deaths had been reported, with U.S. numbers being twenty-nine and three, respectively — I quit worrying about it. But the event had changed my feelings about the company from simple gratitude to admiration. They had not dodged the problem. They had sent me a letter in plain English telling me what was going on and what I could do to protect myself. To be sure, they were required by the FDA to do so, but in situations like this companies can drag their feet or they can tackle it head-on, and Advanced Bionics had done the latter.

And then it was my turn. Van introduced me, and I walked up to the podium and looked into a sea of faces.

Hundreds if not thousands of people have collaborated over decades to build the corporate mind of my ear. They are all now, in an almost literal sense, my ancestors. I have inherited the collective creation of their ideas and thoughts as part of my own body. One can actually *see* their collaboration in the code itself. Part of the snippet of code I presented earlier included the following bit of almost lucid English:

```
/* incr = 3; */
incr = 2;  /* 3-8-2000 based on input from
   Jason Lee and Michael Stone */
```

The /* and */ characters bracket off text that the computer knows it's supposed to ignore. It's there solely for the benefit of the human programmers. Notes, comments, questions. Apparently on March 8, 2000, two people named Jason Lee and Michael Stone persuaded the programmer that the value of *incr* should be 2 instead of 3. But the programmer wasn't quite convinced, for instead of simply making the change, he bracketed off the line *incr = 3* by telling the computer to ignore it. That way, if things went haywire because *incr* was 2, he could easily remember the former value and restore it.

No doubt e-mails and phone calls went in various directions over the value of *incr*. The programmer and Jason Lee were at Advanced Bionics in California, and Michael Stone was on the other side of the world, at the Department of Experimental Psychology in Cambridge, England. Lee and Stone had coauthored a paper on this very programming issue a year before, so they knew each other across all those miles. When I read the code, I could sense the old echoes of their conversations. I knew that I could hear *just so* because the three of them had decided together, after some debate, that *incr* should be 2.

Here, in this room, were many of the people who had made painstaking decisions like these. Not all of them, not the university scientists, not the engineers at Cochlear and Med-El who broke so much of the ground Advanced Bionics has trod, not the people who had retired or died by now. Not Graeme Clark nor Rod Saunders, who are in Australia, nor George Watson nor Michael

Pierschalla, who are in the grave. But many of them were here. There was Logan Palmer, designer of the microprocessors in my head; there was Mike Faltys, chief engineer; there was Tracey Kruger, who had upgraded me to Hi-Res; and there was Leo Litvak, smiling benignly at me from whatever ineffable realm of spirit or code he happened to be inhabiting at the moment.

"I went deaf on July 7, 2001, at ten-thirty in the morning," I began, and the story unfolded from there. I told them what it was like to grow up without language. I tried to explain what the world sounded like the day of my activation, using a page from Bettelheim's article about Joey as a prop, with half the letters whited out. I talked about visiting Summit Speech School and seeing the children there pronounce *Pennsylvania* perfectly and chatter with their parents. They would not have to go through the things I did; for many of them, profound deafness would be merely an *inconvenience.* As I painted a picture of the school in words for them, to my shock I felt tears starting to gather in the corners of my eyes.

I *never* cry, and here I was about to do it in front of 150 people. I took a deep breath and sighed to compose myself. I talked some more, then opened the floor for questions.

It was a hell of a risk. Big echoing room, with people a hundred feet away from me. Finally a young man, mercifully near the front of the room, raised his hand and asked me what considerations were uppermost in my mind as I weighed which implant to get.

"I'll tell you, shopping for a new ear is a very strange experience," I said, and a light ripple of laughter went up. Then I answered the question. "Upgrade potential," I said crisply. "That was *the* main consideration. My mom said to me, 'Mike, don't focus on the hardware. Focus on the software. Focus not just on what it can do now, but on what it may be able to do in the future.'"

A hand went up in the middle of the room, a slender Indian-looking fellow who I would find out afterward was a native of Sri Lanka. I nodded at him, and then I realized that I might be in trouble. But I understood him with little effort, pulling in more than enough of his phonemes to construct his meaning. What new products would I like to see, he wanted to know, as a user?

"Wish list," I said thoughtfully, looking off into the distance to collect my ideas. I launched into a little disquisition on what I wanted to see in microphone design. Microphone design and placement aren't glamorous, I said, but it made a huge difference. I told them about the chest-microphone trick Doug Lynch taught me. Then half a dozen hands went up and the questions flooded in. I will never forget that day, their eager alert faces, the effortless back-and-forth of question and answer and follow-up, the laughter that periodically went up in gentle phase-coded waves.

In group therapy almost a decade earlier, I had been proud of extending my range to fifteen feet. Here my range was seventy-five feet, one hundred. Were it some other crowd, I might not have done as well. But I knew these people, they had rebuilt me; in every single millisecond their voices were passing through the software they themselves had crafted, and my neurons had physically reshaped themselves in response to the curve and arc of their thoughts. We were united by a common fascination, a common enterprise. They had begun to feel — could I dare to think it? — like *friends.* In all the places I had ever been in my whole life, this place, here, now, felt the most like home.

11. The Technologies of Human Potential

EMILY: Do any human beings ever realize life while they live it — every, every minute?

STAGE MANAGER: No. (pause) The saints and poets, maybe they do, some.

— THORNTON WILDER, *Our Town*

FRESHLY FALLEN SNOW: two athletes in ski gear, racing downhill at high speed.

One of them has the very latest skis, a pair made with expensive composites. He's sixteen, immortal, intoxicated by pure speed. The other one is thirty-five and his skis are five years old, a little heavier, a little scratched up. But he knows how to read the snow, knows exactly what his skis can and can't do, knows his own strengths and limitations. Who's going to win?

I'd put my money on the older guy.

The ski gear's important, but it's only one factor among many. It is often the athlete with the better *mind* that wins. Better emotions, too: an ability to focus on the task unclouded by fear or guilt or self-consciousness.

A few weeks after I was activated, I realized that I had to become an athlete of perception. I had to learn to glide over the soundstream like a skier over bumpy snow, to assemble meanings out of phonemes like a juggler keeping ten balls in the air. Fifty thousand dollars had just been spent on me, but it wasn't the end of my reconstruction. It was just the beginning. But with all that our civilization knows about human performance, you'd think I would have coaches, training programs, multimedia CD-ROMs, the works. Wrong. No formal training of any kind was offered to me during those tumultuous and difficult months after activation.

It's not that I lacked support. In many ways I had excellent preparation and support for the task of learning to hear again, from my childhood training to group therapy to Becky's endless patience in fitting me with map after map.

It's not that there weren't resources out there, either. There are speech therapists aplenty, and the House Ear Institute in L.A. has developed a computerized training system to help cochlear implant users learn to recognize vowels and consonants. All three implant companies have programs intended to pair up experienced users with new users, as coaches. But what was lacking was an institutional structure that put those resources together for me and walked me through using them: there was no Cochlear Implant 101. What "training" I had I scrounged up myself from books on tape and National Public Radio.

The raw material for Cochlear Implant 101 is out there. What's missing is an ethos of human performance similar to that taken for granted in sport. But does it really matter? After all, I *did* learn to hear all over again, on my own.

I think it does matter — and here's why. In group therapy, I learned that I could hear people considerably better with *no changes at all* to my hardware or software. I think that with the right training I would have adapted faster, and reached a higher performance level than I'm at now. The fact that I can use a telephone is a wonder of twenty-first-century engineering, but I still struggle to hear in crowds. Do I *have* to struggle? Can I do better?

Perhaps, with the right training. Here's an example of what even a little training did for me. In May 2004, I took a hearing test designed to measure how well I could recognize vowel sounds. (I was again volunteering myself as a guinea pig.) In this test the computer spoke a word beginning with *b* and ending with *t* and I had to decide whether it was *beet, bit, bat, bite, boot,* or any other of about twenty choices. The test would have been easy but for the fact that the vowel was electronically adjusted so that it was always the same duration. When *beet* is no longer than *bit,* the only way to tell them apart is by the pitch of the vowel sound. Normally hearing people will ace the test, but since frequency discrimination is one of the implant's weakest points, the test is very difficult for people like me. I'd taken it several times before, and my scores were usually in the 30 percent range.

Which made me mad. How could I not be able to distinguish between *bet* and *bit?* How hard could an *eh* sound be? So this time I started sneaking looks at the data set after each run, looking for my characteristic errors. I soon discovered that whenever it said *bit,* I usually thought it was *bet.* But when it actually said *bet,* I usually got it right. *Aha.* I started listening extra closely every time I thought I was hearing *bet,* listening for that oh-so-subtle difference that would let me tell whether it was actually *bit. You neurons, you sort it out in there.* As the runs went on, I got better and better at it. My score on the last run was 60 percent.

Training makes an *enormous* difference. Research in neurobiology is showing that the right kind of training has directly measurable effects on people's brains. According to studies in 2002 and 2004, the auditory cortex of musicians is 130 percent larger than that of nonmusicians, and children exposed to music early in life show auditory brain activity comparable to children three years older who had not been exposed. It makes a difference. So does learning to feel a sense of connection with other human beings, and having a wholeness of spirit, an unclouded mind. Absent those things, you can outfit people with cyborg technologies at great cost, but they'll fail to make the most of them. In fact, I would be willing to bet that people with perfectly ordinary bodies but excellent training will often outperform them.

Put this way, the point seems almost too obvious to mention. Everyone knows that the best gear in the world won't make an inexperienced skier into a champion. But what we know with regard to sports we seem to forget with technology. I was given the most sophisticated cyborg device in existence and essentially told, "Here. *You* figure out how to use it."

Perhaps it's because sports have been around for thousands of years, while cyborg technologies are extremely new. There's an infatuation with them that hasn't yet been tempered by reality and experience. My own experience has profoundly changed my perspective on Hollywood productions such as *Star Trek* and *Robocop,* which now strike me as shallow and naive, more akin to superhero fantasies than credible visions of the future. It seems be a widespread assumption that cyborg technologies will in themselves lead to expanded human capabilities. I think that's unrealistic. Consider the fact that my real-world ability to understand speech in noise, so far as I can tell, is about the same — perhaps somewhat better — than it was with hearing aids, even though the method of delivering sound to my brain has changed profoundly. Things *sound* different, but my *performance* is about the same. Before going completely deaf, I was what most audiologists would call a borderline case, someone whose aided hearing performance was already approximately equivalent to what I could expect from an implant. Even so, I probably get more total information from the implant, because it triggers nerve endings that hadn't had hair cells before. But I'm limited by having an auditory cortex that's not developed enough to *use* the additional information. Take an example: at a conference in 2003, while I was walking across a plaza full of people talking and eating, someone ran up to me from behind. "I was calling your name, but you didn't hear me," she said. And then I realized: I *had* heard her! I hadn't turned around because I didn't *believe* I could be hearing someone calling my name amid such noise. The phoneme "Mike" had vaguely registered in my mind, but I'd ignored it. Experiences like that give me the strong feeling that the limiting factor in my hearing is my *brain,* not the technology.

That's why I'm skeptical of the apparently widespread belief that installing new hardware in the body will by itself expand human powers. Take, for example, one of Kevin Warwick's predictions in his book *I, Cyborg*. He writes, "Human communication is on the verge of a complete overhaul. We will shortly make much more use of the technology that can send and receive millions of messages, in parallel, with zero error. We will interface with machines through thought signals. We will become nodes on a techno-network. We will be able to communicate with other humans merely by thinking to each other. Speech, as we know it, may well become obsolete."

There are so many problematic claims in these six sentences that it's hard to know where to begin in discussing them. First, let me point out that neural technologies are *nowhere near* to being sophisticated enough to make this scenario possible. Consider my own ear. My implant gives me sixteen channels of auditory information, whereas a normal ear delivers the equivalent of thousands. Replacing the ear with a metal/ceramic/silicon substitute is akin to fixing a spider web with yarn. This is no insult to the engineers, whose work is brilliant. It is rather a recognition of how exquisitely complex and integrated a normally functioning body is, and how little of it we still understand. And that's just the *ear*. We are a long way from understanding our own brains well enough to implant devices in them to enhance our mental functioning.

It's disconcerting that Kevin Warwick in particular should be making such claims, because he himself has done significant research in neural interfaces. He implanted an electrode array in his wrist that could pick up impulses from his median nerve. That allowed him to control external devices such as a three-fingered robot hand and a power wheelchair. He also put a similar electrode array in his wife's wrist so that the computer could pick up nerve impulses from him and pass them along to her. When Warwick moved his hand, his wife felt a sensation in her own. It went both ways, so they could signal back and forth.

That's impressive work. But one can't extrapolate from controlling a wheelchair to predicting that "speech, as we know it, may well become obsolete." The median nerve in the wrist is one thing, the brain is quite another. One would have to install a huge number of electrodes directly in the brain to pick up the neural activity corresponding to language. Interpreting the resulting data — or even just passing it on to another brain — would require an extraordinary amount of filtering and processing. At this point, it's in the realm of science fiction, not science fact.

Warwick also suggests that cyborg technologies can enhance intelligence as well as communication. He writes, "With the interlinking of human and machine brains, even in a relatively limited way, it should be possible, within the next fifteen years, to upgrade memory, improve mathematical capabilities and increase considerably one's knowledge base. When linked to the network, a cyborg has the potential for an intelligence way beyond that of a standalone human." Once again, I have doubts about technical feasibility. But more than that, the brain isn't a computer that can be upgraded by plugging modules into it. It's an organ that evolved over millions of years to solve problems extremely specific to daily life: finding food, recognizing kin and predators, building tools, and so on. One cannot simply add new capabilities to it such as the ability to hold more than seven items in working memory or solve differential equations. If technology is ever developed that can significantly change brain functioning, it will be necessary to educate its users, intensively, in how to make use of whatever new capabilities it makes possible. As we now know, it's possible to reshape the brain's neural wiring with carefully designed exercises. Developing such training in conjunction with neural technologies will be indispensable.

To be sure, cyborg technologies may soon be able to restore *lost* mental capabilities to some extent. For that, research such as Warwick's is unquestionably valuable. A company called Cyberkinetics is designing "brain implant" chips that may be able to pick up neural signals and translate them into commands that will move artificial limbs. Similar work is being done by Duke University's Miguel Nicolelis, who has trained monkeys to move artificial arms by mental signals — that is, by thinking. But these technologies are only for people with serious medical conditions. Warwick consistently neglects this important qualification. Upon having used his implant to pilot an electric wheelchair he comments, "I told everyone that this would ultimately mean, in the future, we should be able to drive a car around by picking up the signals directly from the brain, and change direction just by thinking about it, right, left, and so on." For disabled people, this is an exciting prospect. But the rest of us already *do* drive with signals from our brains, picked up and executed perfectly by our arms and legs.

Warwick might respond that having direct nervous control over an automobile would let us drive it better, since we wouldn't have to move around our heavy meat arms and legs. But then issues of practicality and safety come into play. Andy Clark and Gregory Stock have both argued that for the vast majority of people, fyborg ("functional cyborg") technologies are far cheaper and safer than cyborg technologies. In science fiction, cyborgs are superheroes. But in real life, cyborg body parts need frequent tinkering and constant battery changes, and they are never as good as the natural organs they replace. I suppose you *could,* if you had the requisite millions of dollars, build a bionic eye that let its user see in the infrared, but it would not be as good as the eye it replaced, and you could also simply wear infrared goggles at a fraction of the cost and zero surgical risk.

Whenever I read enthusiastic predictions about the benefits of implantable computer technology, I think of a patient whom I'll call Beth, who had the same surgeon, the same implant, the same audiologist, and the same software as I did, but with totally different results. She'd lost her hearing gradually, starting in her fifties. Hopes were high for her success, because she had all the right factors: normal hearing for much of her life, longtime stimulation of her auditory system with hearing aids, high intelligence, excellent speech. Beth's surgery and activation seemed to go well, but when I asked her how she was doing a few weeks later, she sighed and looked off into the distance before answering. Her face said: maybe it's working, but I can't say I *like* it.

Nine months after her activation, it was clear that she was not becoming a successful user. She told me that what she heard was muddy, hollow, and indistinct. I had to speak to her almost as slowly and carefully as before her implant surgery, and she had the same tense, concentrated look as before on her face as she struggled to listen to me. Worse than that, she had an endless succession of hardware problems. Incredibly, *six* processors in a row failed on her. One by one they would stop booting up, or work intermittently.

Suspicion naturally alighted on the implant itself. But diagnostic x-rays showed that the electrode array was correctly positioned, and Advanced Bionics tested her several times without finding anything wrong with the electronics. I was able to personally confirm that some of her processors were indeed not working correctly by trying them on myself. (Our maps were quite similar.) It seemed almost as if healthy processors gave up and died when they got near her.

It's hard enough to learn to use a cochlear implant with a reliable processor. With each setback she fell further and further behind and got more and more discouraged. When Advanced Bionics released Hi-Res, she got it loaded into her processor, hoping it might help. Her processors did stop breaking, to everyone's relief. However, her hearing didn't improve. If anything, a year later she was doing worse on Hi-Res than on SAS.

I began describing Beth's predicament to various scientists and engineers, hoping that someone would have the magic key to unlock her ear. Everyone had a different theory. One person suggested that it could be some subtle kind of failure in the device, undetectable by the diagnostic tests. Another opined that perhaps she had poor nerve survival in that ear. Still another thought she might be relying too much on her unimplanted ear so that her brain wasn't developing the ability to use the implant.

There might, in fact, be no single cause. So many factors contribute to a person's outcome that understanding their interaction is almost impossible. In the end, Beth's poor results are a mystery. After decades of research and development such outcomes are rare, but they are not unheard of. So now, whenever I hear blithe predictions that in the future bionic implants of various kinds will be nearly universal, I think of Beth, whose life is a testament to the fact that the human body is far from a fully solved problem. In many ways biomedical engineers are still sorcerers' apprentices, chanting half-understood incantations and hoping for the best.

It's possible, of course, that technological advances will address these limitations. My perspective is undoubtedly colored by my own experience with present-day cyborg technologies, whose limitations are a daily fact of my life. But if I had to predict what technologies would have the most impact on normal, nondisabled bodies in the long run, I would put my money on ones that subtly change the body from within, on a cellular level, rather than cutting it open and overriding it: pharmaceuticals, genetic engineering, nanotechnology.

While I'm skeptical of Warwick's predictions, of course I can't say they're not going to happen. How could I, living in a body that many experts had believed to be impossible? (In his memoir of developing the Nucleus 24 cochlear implant, Graeme Clark lists five frequently mentioned obstacles that many experts had considered insuperable.) My biggest disagreement with Warwick is that he speaks of the human body as if it were as impersonal and upgradeable as a desktop computer. It is not. Rebuilding human beings requires the resources and perspectives of an entire society, not just engineers. What about "overhauling human communication" by teaching people how to listen and negotiate? What about "improving mathematical capabilities" by halving the size of math classes and doubling teachers' salaries? It's culture and education that make us human and humane, not the machines we implant in our bodies.

Frank Herbert's *Dune* fascinates me because it's a vision of a society that focuses on the mind the way ours focuses on the body. It's got serious limitations — the world of *Dune* is a feudal theocracy — but in many ways, it's got the right idea. *Mentats* are trained from childhood to absorb vast quantities of information and synthesize it while advising rulers and planning military campaigns. Secretaries record verbatim transcripts of meetings in their heads. Soldiers and religious leaders are trained to consciously regulate their own body processes and develop extraordinary sensitivity to the environment around them. One character slows her metabolism down to almost nothing to survive being trapped in an avalanche, and identifies most of a village's industries simply by sniffing the air.

Fiction? It doesn't have to be. Monks of certain sects can regulate their body temperature, heart rate, and other physiological processes with extraordinary precision, and Islamic scholars routinely memorize the entire Koran. In medieval times, a skilled troubadour needed to hear a long poem recited only three times to commit the entire thing to memory; university teachers were said to be able to repeat a hundred lines of text after hearing it recited only once. What should be surprising is not their achievements but the fact that such achievements are now so rare. Mnemonic techniques such as the "memory palace," where people memorized information by situating it in a visualized physical space, have been known for hundreds if not thousands of years.

While some particular technologies of human performance — "mnemotechnics," as Francis Yates called them — have become irrelevant (who needs to memorize text?), the *idea* of mnemotechnics should be revived. If technology can indeed enlarge human capabilities, people will need intensive training to use those capabilities. They will need to become athletes of perception, downhill skiers of cognition, craftsmen of communication. Put *Dune* and *I, Cyborg* together, and you begin to get a vision of a world where technology is used humanely to make better human beings.

When I think of the future of human potential in a hypertechnological age, I imagine a generation of people who have been educated to focus intensely on the world of matter and spirit, while also using powerful tools for mediating their perception of reality.

They will bond with machines, but they will not be addicted to them. They will analyze while looking at art, and laugh while reading computer code. They will make exquisite use of floods of information, while not allowing themselves to be stunned into passivity. They will know how to make choices. They will know how to sift, discriminate, sense, judge, and intuit. They will know how to speak, and how to listen. Above all, they will know how to love.

I would name this kind of human *Homo faber,* the artistic human, the creating and self-creating human. *Homo faber* is inherently a creature of technology, because there could be no art without pencils and paper, paintbrushes, guitars, saxophones, and word processors. (If you think pencils and paper aren't technologies, try making them yourself.) *Homo faber* is a person who achieves a deeper connection to the world with technology than he or she could have without it.

Homo faber will know better than to let technology undermine community. In *Bowling Alone,* Robert Putnam carefully examines various social factors in an attempt to locate the core causes of community decline. It turns out that the single biggest culprit is television. Putnam estimates that television *alone* accounts for about 25 percent of the decline, far more than any other single factor. "Dependence on television for entertainment is not merely *a* significant predictor of civic disengagement," Putnam writes. "It is the *single most consistent predictor* that I have discovered." My own critique of television is that *it* constructs *you;* its way of feeding you stimulation turns you into a couch potato. Instead, *Homo faber* would gravitate toward technologies which encourage *self*-construction.

An encouraging attitude toward technology can be found in Steve Mann's book about how computer technologies can be used to mediate perception. As mentioned earlier, Mann has developed wearable computers with tiny monitors constantly positioned in front of one eye. I must admit that until I read Mann's book, I thought his wearable computer gear made him look embarrassingly geeky. But his goal is to enable people to live in environments of their own choosing, rather than in ones that governments or corporations choose for them:

> It may seem contrary to intuition that freedom is to be found in such a seemingly intrusive imposition as a grid mediating your contact with the world. Yet, as someone who lives in MR [Mediated Reality] every day, I feel like I've discovered a way to live that returns my humanity to me . . . The supposed freedom we have in democratic society is severely limited by our inability to walk down a street without breathing in the exhaust from thousands of cars while exposing our minds to countless advertising images (three thousand per day for the average citizen of the United States). As Greil Marcus so succinctly realizes, a reality is already imposed on us. The challenge now is to make that reality subjective, to figure out how to use technology to assert our right to individual and community realities . . .

In giving people the ability to mediate reality on their own terms, Mann believes that he is offering them the freedom to think and act on their own terms. He writes, "The solution will be to find ways to improve our ability to process and consume and decide what information should reach us on an individual basis." I have concerns about Mann's approach: is it really progress to have a computer decide what we will see, instead of teaching people to recognize media manipulation and helping them focus their attention on the things that truly matter to them? Nonetheless, in focusing on self-construction and individual choice, Mann is asking the right questions and exploring possible answers with admirable thoroughness. My cochlear implant gave me the opportunity to reconstruct myself. My struggles with it were strongly related to the fact that it *did* impose a premade conception of reality on me to some extent. One of the things I wished for most dearly was more control over the software's parameters. I yearned to be able to tinker with it — and myself — on a more fundamental level than the processor's three dials allowed.

How close are we to becoming *Homo faber,* as a species? Not close at all, I think. It takes far more than putting technology onto, or into, people's bodies. It takes lifetimes of education and training, and the creation of a society secure and confident enough to understand that true power comes from communication and understanding, rather than heavy weaponry.

I think my experience with the computer in my skull has given me an inkling of what it must be like to be *Homo faber,* but only an inkling. I spent the first forty-six months of my life deaf, and many more years after that addicted to the computer. The logic of the incantation has penetrated both my body and soul. Sometimes I connect deeply with people. More often I struggle to connect, and fail. The one hundred and forty thousand transistors in my skull give me sound, but they cannot make me *listen.* It's only when I listen that my cyborg technologies make me a better human being.

12. Mike 2.0

I came to see the damage that was done
and the treasures that prevail.

— ADRIENNE RICH, "Diving into the Wreck" (1973)

JULY 2004. Three years have gone by since I went deaf. It is getting harder and harder to describe what hearing through a cochlear implant sounds like, for my memories of life with hearing aids are receding into the past. But my hearing is getting better and better. I hadn't realized *how* much better until Becky compiled my scores on the HINT +5dB test over time. HINT stands for "Hearing in Noise Test," in which sentences are spoken against a background of white noise. The "+5dB" means that the sentences are only five decibels louder than the noise. The lower the number, the tougher the test. In the HINT +0dB test the sentences are the same volume as the noise, making it a pure pattern recognition test. A visual analogue of what the tests sound like would look something like this:

No noise	The boy walked the dog.
HINT +10dB	The boy walked the dog.
HINT +5dB	The boy walked the dog.
HINT +0dB	The boy walked the dog.

Normally hearing people would score close to 100 percent on all of these tests, but for hearing-impaired people they are very difficult. The first time I took the HINT +5dB test in January 2002, three months post-activation, I thought to myself, "This is impossible. Complete hash. I'll never score well on *this* test." My score was 17 percent. But this spring I sailed through it. Becky put together my scores over time:

January 2002	17%
February 2003	39%
April 2004	70%

A score of 70 percent would be bad news for a normally hearing person. But for a totally deaf man, it's like a dog getting a C in algebra.

That's just the testing booth, though. What matters is the real world. When I saw *The Fellowship of the Ring* in the theater in 2001, I understood very little of the dialogue. In 2004, watching *The Return of the King*, I understood *all* of the dialogue. *All* of it. A wonder! A wonder!

It's new software at work. In 2001, I had eight channels of auditory input and a pulse rate that wasn't very well suited to my neural physiology. In 2004, I have sixteen channels and a pulse rate that may be sending more information to my brain.

It's neural plasticity at work. Prodded by the implant's electrical stimulation, my auditory cortex has slowly reshaped itself by growing new dendritic connections every which way. Three years after going deaf I have a differently wired brain, molded and shaped in the computer's image.

It's emotional growth at work. I am a better human being now, friendlier and more tolerant, with less internal static clouding my ability to hear not just what people *say* but what people *mean*.

The dizziness, and also the baffling fluctuations in my hearing, have diminished to the point where they no longer bother me. My visual system has picked up the slack so well that I can do anything I could before, except stand on one foot with my eyes closed. Eyes open, it's easy. Close my eyes, and in a few seconds I start wobbling.

The hermetically sealed gyroscopes of my ears are damaged, but to compensate I have learned to supplement my navigation through the world with the compasses of my eyes.

There are compensations for being expelled from the Garden. No single story controls my reality, but I am liberated to make up *stories.* Recently I dreamed that I was in a theater where people held up their hands so that their shadows would be cast onto the screen. (It was, now that I think back on it, a twenty-first-century version of Plato's cave.) A computer would detect the silhouette of your hand and superimpose a large animated hand in its place, a purple polka-dotted one for example, or a scaly eagle's talon, which was still "yours" because it perfectly matched your movements. You never knew what you would get when you held up your hand, and children were shouting in delight and adults were laughing to see the wonderfully jumbled forest of monstrous hands waving and flapping on the screen.

And then the scene shifted, and we could see the monsters themselves full-bodied on the stage, the kind that Maurice Sendak would draw, projected by the computer in three dimensions. When you pointed at one it would stretch right up to you to grin hello, and it was both scary and exciting to see those gruff, benign faces responding so directly to your finger. The sheer *responsiveness* of the system was thrilling. You pointed, it came right up to you. How, I wondered, did the computer decide what to do when two people pointed to the same monster? Did it choose one of them at random? Did both people somehow see the monster coming up to them? Programmer that I was, I worried about this problem, but I knew that these monsters and the computer giving life to them were not to be feared; they were allies and friends. Then I stood up and floated effortlessly into the air, gliding around the theater above the seats. I am having dreams of levitation and flying far more often than I used to. It may be because my body no longer feels fully solid and grounded. My waking life is a computer's dream of reality, and my body feels ethereally light. I now require a horizon to stand with two feet squarely upon the earth. In the darkness of sleep it takes only a little nudge now, a step and a lift, for my body to take flight.

Simply putting the implant in my skull did not in itself trigger all the ways I've changed and grown. I chose to make the most of the experience, the way a surfer takes advantage of a wave. Going deaf is a kind of death, but by the grace of technology I have been able to go through the experience and emerge, both intact and different, on the other side.

In May 2004, I'd noticed that the bone around the implant seemed to have changed. There was a sort of dip in my skull next to the rounded end that my fingers hadn't felt before. I grew a little worried: maybe the bone around the implant was *eroding?* I visualized the ceramic casing suddenly sliding backward out of its countersunk hollow in my skull, unreeling the electrode array out of my cochlea like a snapped rubber band. I made an appointment. Dr. Roberson thoughtfully probed the area with his fingers, pushing and tugging the implant much more firmly than I would ever dare to. I felt a brief thrill of fright: What if it moved, like a tooth coming loose? But in a moment he had me sit up. "It's fine, Mike," he told me. "It's normal for the area to change a little bit over time. I gave it a good tug and it's solidly anchored. The bone's grown around it and locked it into place. In fact, if I wanted to remove it now, I'd have to drill it out of your skull."

So it's truly part of me now. My hearing tests prove that my little computer and I have adapted beautifully to each other, making us a *cybernetic organism.* My hearing aids had just shouted at me. If I pulled them out they whistled stupidly, picking up their own output and reamplifying it until it was ratcheted up to a scream. (It's the same as the squeal that happens when a microphone is placed too close to the speakers in an auditorium: *feedback.*) But the little green LED on my processor turns red and begins blinking when the headpiece falls off. That's because it's no longer receiving the periodic "I am here" status reports radioed to it from the circuitry in my skull. *My processor knows when it is not attached to me.* That makes us a system, rather than just a prosthesis and a human being latched together. My processor feels "lonely," in its dim electronic way, when I'm not around.

I now know how to collaborate with a computer to construct a world. In that, my experience contradicts what some critics of technology might have predicted. In his book *Readings,* Sven Birkerts argues that technology alienates people from the natural rhythms of life and from each other. Instead of knowing the world through direct sense-experience, Birkerts suggests, we increasingly experience it through technological devices. "We have put between ourselves and the natural world so many layers of signals, noises, devices, and habits that the chance for connection is very limited," he writes.

I don't dispute that this may be true — witness television as the prime example. But I also note that I should be more susceptible to this kind of alienation than almost anyone, because the computer mediates my perception of the world to an unprecedented degree. My auditory world does not even *exist* without the computer. Yet I feel more connected to the world post-activation, rather than less. Obviously, part of the reason is that the computer lets me hear; there's nothing more isolating than deafness. But there's more to it than that. What saved me from alienation was not just being able to hear again, but also being forced to construct my world rather than simply taking it as a given. In retrospect, I see it as a blessing that I had two kinds of software to choose from, SAS and CIS. At the time it made an already confusing experience even more so, but being able to compare them, and work with Becky to customize their parameters, encouraged me to think about my hearing in terms of choice rather than simple adaptation. Which versions of the world sounded better? Which ones gave me better performance? I could hardly be alienated from the world, for it was a world I had helped to construct.

CIS and SAS have now been phased out in favor of Hi-Res, not just because it is supposed to be better, but also because audiologists simply don't have the time to fit all of their patients with two different kinds of software. While I grant the clinical necessity of it, I am rather sorry to see SAS and CIS go, because now patients will have only one version of reality to choose from. All too often, progress entails taking two steps forward and one backward.

I was saved from alienation in another way as well. Each day when I get dressed, I have a choice between two versions of the processor. One is the small box I wear on my hip with a wire running under my shirt to the headpiece. The other is the one that looks like a hearing aid, with a short cable running to the headpiece. The latter is a lot easier to put on, and it works just as well. Better, in fact, because it has a clever microphone design that uses the outer ear as a funnel to collect sound. But I usually choose to wear the box on my hip. The reason? *It doesn't look like a hearing aid.* Few people know *what* the heck it is, and I find that wonderfully liberating. It frees me from all the cultural baggage that hearing aids carry. When people see hearing aids, all sorts of assumptions come into play about the wearers: that they are slow, that they have to be shouted at, that they are old. But when I'm wearing a simple disk behind my ear with a thin cable disappearing under my shirt, I leap wholly outside the space of those assumptions. After explaining the implant to people — I get a kick out of pulling the headpiece off and demonstrating that its magnet is strong enough to hold forks and key rings — I sometimes ask them what they thought it was. I've gotten answers like these:

"I thought it might be a chemo dispenser, but people on chemotherapy don't usually do five-mile hikes."

"I thought it was a cell phone earbud."

"Uh . . . I thought you had something stuck in your hair."

"I thought it was where you put the gas in." (We both started laughing.)

"I thought it was a Secret Service thing, but you don't *look* Secret Service."

No one could ever mistake me for being Secret Service. But with the belt-worn version of the implant, I can define myself on my own terms, not other people's. I have more freedom now to shape the way people perceive me, and to choose how I want to perceive myself.

In the movie *Star Trek: Nemesis,* there is a scene where Data inserts a computer jack behind his ear in order to download data from another android. (An android — to get technical about it — is a robot that looks especially like a human being.) The point of such scenes is to evoke the kind of shiver that comes from seeing boundaries transgressed, familiar assumptions violated. Before my surgery, one of the things that most frightened me was knowing that the sheer weirdness of latching a data terminal onto my skull would, at some point, become normal, a casual part of my daily life. The feeling of being normal again: *that* would signify that I had truly changed. The prospect had made me pull the sheets over my head and curl up into a ball.

But I felt no sense of weirdness as I watched Data go through the process. The data terminal was exactly where the headpiece of a cochlear implant goes, so Data's hand motion to put the jack in place was utterly familiar. Data and his twin sat back to back, the computer between them as intermediary, and this too was familiar. Many times audiologists have plugged my headpiece directly into their laptops, running my ear out of an ordinary Pentium rather than the specialized hardware of my processor. The scene seemed so unremarkable as to be hardly worth filming. And *that* was strange. To watch something intended to be so weird, and to find it so ordinary.

Here in the dark damaged wood of my destroyed inner ear, approaching the middle of my life, I have accounted for my losses. But against them I have accounted for my gains as well. I've had the ambiguous privilege of having a story to tell. To the Greeks blindness was a brutal gift from the gods, enabling the victim to become a singer of tales. Deafness can be that kind of gift, too. I gripe about cell phone reception like everyone else, but I am well aware that the fact that I *can* gripe is extraordinary, akin to a blind man complaining that newspaper ink smudges his fingers. For thousands of years people have dreamed of making the deaf hear. Only in the last twenty-five years has that become possible, and only in the last five has the technology really taken off. It is now possible to say that if a child's deafness is detected by eighteen months, it may be the least of her problems in life.

To be sure, the implant is a prosthesis, not a cure. When the headpiece falls off or the battery dies, I'm as deaf as ever. And people with cochlear implants don't always realize their potential, as Beth's experience sadly demonstrates. My own performance is still confusingly variable. Sometimes I hear flawlessly, sometimes I struggle. I heard *The Return of the King* perfectly, but when I went to see *Robot Stories* in Berkeley a few months after that, I could understand only scraps of the dialogue. My ability to hear depends on many things, including the acoustics, how alert I am, how much of the context I know, how clearly people speak, and how connected I feel to them. It's like cell phones. Sometimes I get a good signal, sometimes I don't. But on the whole, deafness's power to limit and blight lives is clearly coming to an end.

In his memoir *Deafness*, David Wright considers the question of whether he would want his hearing miraculously restored, and concludes that he would not:

> For I am now, after forty years of what we will term silence, so accommodated to it (like a hermit-crab to its shell) that were the faculty of hearing restored to me tomorrow it would appear as an affliction rather than a benefit . . . the disability has been assimilated to the extent that it is now an integral condition of my existence, like the use of a hand. By the same token the restoration of my hearing, or the loss of my deafness, whichever is the right way of putting it, would be like having that hand cut off.

I have considered the same question, but unlike Wright I would accept the gift of normal hearing without hesitation. *It could happen.* Research progresses apace on ways of regenerating hair cells. Bird ears do it naturally; there's no such thing as a deaf bird. Scientists are now studying bird ears in the hope of reproducing their mechanisms of hair cell regrowth in mammals. It has already been done, to some extent, in guinea pigs and rats. Everyone agrees that the challenges are formidable, but they do not appear to be insuperable.

Maybe someday that research will come to fruition. Perhaps someday when I am in my fifties the implant and its electrode array will be ever so gently removed, and a witches' brew of chemicals and neurotransmitters injected in its place that will, over the next few months, re-grow the garden fields in both of my inner ears. What would that be like, the slow awakening of my ears? What would it be like to have normal hearing? How can I possibly know? But I have lived in so many versions of reality that I have lost count of them; I am familiar with my body changing over and over again. This would be simply the next change, yet another transformative adventure in a life that has had more than its full share of them. For that day, I can be patient.

In the spring of 2004, Laura and I went for a walk in a park to catch up. She was as beautiful as ever. It was bittersweet to see her, for I felt both happiness and longing. The tense set of her shoulders told me all I needed to know about her feelings, but I had to try; it's built into me not to give up. After a while I laid it out once again. I told her how much I thought about her, and how much I admired her questing spirit. "We could make a great couple," I said wistfully, "if we could just get over the chemistry issue."

She said she would think about it. And I knew I had lost, once again.

But I just have to continue being what I am, which is part animal, part computer, all human, and let the species figure out in its own slow time what to do with me. I am making progress in finding a community: my Palm Pilot is now full of the names of writers, artists, agents, editors, scientists, and engineers. Joe Quirk and I often get together over tacos to fuss over manuscripts, plot our careers, and talk about women. I get invited to parties more often now, too, and I feel a happy little burst of surprise and gratitude every time an evite shows up in my inbox.

Maybe I have just a little more of an idea of what love is all about, now. In 1995 I was sitting at the bottom of my apartment's steps in Austin taking in the evening. A white cat with black markings walked by, took a look at me, stopped, and sat on its haunches so it could look me boldly in the eye. *Greetings, human.*

I said, "Hi! Who are you?"

For answer it hopped up on the step beside me. I stroked its fur, which was baby-seal soft. After a few minutes it climbed into my lap, balanced itself carefully on my legs, butted its head against my sternum, and purred so hard I could feel it in my spine.

"*Hiiii,*" I said. I checked its flea collar: no tag.

After a few days in which it came by to visit regularly, I wrote a little note, *What is this cat's name?*, folded it over, carefully stapled it around the flea collar, and let the cat amble off.

A day or two later it was back, with a new note. I detached it and opened it up. *His name is Elvis.*

"Hi, Elvis," I said. He arched his back happily.

I wrote another little note back: *And who owns him?*

The answer came the next day. *My name is Wendy. I live in Building 7.*

In the meantime Elvis had discovered that I had a couch, a bed, and food in the kitchen. We'd play, and he'd get so wildly excited that he would take a flying leap off the couch, bank off the hallway to the bedroom (all four paws hitting the wall), tumble onto my bed, and then run back into the living room. I hated to kick him out so that he would go back to Wendy. I'd try to lure him out the door with a string and he'd take it in his teeth and try to pull me back into the apartment. Soon he'd settled in, spending most of his nights curled up at the foot of my bed.

A few more notes went back and forth on Elvis's flea collar. Wendy and I were communicating by cat. I got her apartment number and phone. It had the makings of *such* a perfect story to tell at a wedding. But she was curiously elusive. I called and spoke to her once or twice, but somehow we never met in person.

One day I went to knock on Wendy's door — she was never home — and discovered that the apartment was empty. Even the window shades were gone. I ran over to the rental office. "What happened to Wendy in apartment 723?" I panted.

Gone. No forwarding address. Not even a goodbye note on his flea collar.

But Elvis was sitting at the foot of my steps.

Yes! Yes!! The very next day I took him to the vet for shots and bought him a handsome collar, a real one. Its tag had *my* phone number on it.

Nine years later Elvis is still my cat, and he still sits in my lap and bumps his head against my chest and purrs. One of the reasons I love him so dearly is because he decided he wanted to be my cat. They say that's the way love works — that it finds you when you're not looking. I've never understood that, but I have to admit it worked in this case. Maybe I just have to sit in a place where enough of the world goes by to get a good look at me.

At 70 percent, my HINT +5dB scores are so spectacular that I can do almost anything I want in life except learn to play the flute, and maybe someday I will be able to do that, too. In October 2004, I donate half my books to the library, casting off the apparatus of grad school. *Shakespeare and the Popular Voice* — gone. *Surprised by Sin: The Reader in "Paradise Lost"* — gone. Tossed back into the ecosystem of words. I finish paying off my car loan, my student loan, and my credit cards. Debt, zero. Light to the ground, light on my toes. Life is diluted in the suburbs of Silicon Valley, too white, too complacent, too wealthy. I feel like an alien in its bland neighborhoods and office parks, lost in its cash nexus and its obsessions with building beautiful machines. But in the streets of San Francisco, forty minutes north, my little implanted computer and I fit right in. Learning of the green world what is my place. The city's steep sidewalks contain people of all shapes and sizes, counter, original, spare, strange. Perhaps my love will find me there, without tags on her collar. Time to find a little one-bedroom apartment with a backyard where Elvis can feel the sun on his face and the grass on his paws, in a neighborhood where I can just walk out my door and encounter the world whole and full. Rebuilt.

APPENDIX

NOTES

BIBLIOGRAPHY

ACKNOWLEDGMENTS

INDEX

APPENDIX

1,113,636 Bits per Second

Thus I too must praise out of a quiet ear
The great creation to which I owe I am
My grief and my love.

— DAVID WRIGHT, *Monologue of a Deaf Man*

The cochlea operates as a short-term Fourier analyzer separating complex acoustic signals into their frequency components.

— ALAN R. PALMER

"Good m —"

Okay, stop time.

A falling acorn hangs suspended in the air. A waved hand stays outstretched in a cosmic *stop* gesture. A security gate halts at a thirty-degree angle, the guard's nod to an incoming driver frozen into waxen immobility.

Cheryl, my department's administrative assistant, is in the middle of saying *good morning* to me as I walk by her office on the way to my own. Now she's frozen too, her lips pursed in an *O* shape, her mouth preparing to launch the long *awww* sound in m*o*rning into the air.

Now let's start up time again, but very, very slowly, letting it tick by one millisecond at a time while we watch the *O* in m*o*rning make its way from Cheryl's lips to my brain. As she exhales to aspirate the vowel, the force of her breath crowds the air molecules in front of her face. Those molecules don't really go anywhere; what they do is bump into the molecules next to them, passing the shock wave along and then placidly resuming their normal business. If you have ever picked up one of the end balls of that desk toy with five hanging balls and let it fall against the next one, you know what happens: the three middle balls barely budge, while the ball on the other end goes flying. So it is with air molecules, except there is no last air molecule to go zooming off. The shock wave simply proceeds through the air, jostling trillions of molecules just a little bit as it travels, until their combined resistance makes it dissipate.

The shock wave travels about 1.1 feet every thousandth of a second, or millisecond. (In human terms, this is 760 miles per hour, the speed of sound at sea level.) In our new temporal perspective we can see it jostling ever more air molecules as it radiates outward in an expanding sphere. And it *is* a sphere; we tend to think of sound as proceeding in straight lines from source to ear, but in fact the waves go in every direction simultaneously. This means that the energy of the sound wave drops off steeply as the sphere grows. When its radius is two feet, it has four times the surface area it had at one foot. By the time the third millisecond has gone by, it will have nine times the surface area; at the fourth, sixteen times. That's a lot more air molecules to jostle, and sound volume drops proportionately as the energy gets spread out. Cheryl's voice, heard four feet away, is sixteen times softer than it was coming out of her mouth.

By the time the expanding sphere reaches me, ten feet away and nine milliseconds later, the loudness of Cheryl's voice has dropped to one-hundredth of what it was coming out of her mouth. It's still quite audible, which is something of a surprise given how much energy has been lost. We will come back to this point in a moment, because it is extremely important for understanding how both cochlear implants and normal ears work. For now, however, let us content ourselves with seeing what happens when the sound hits the microphone of my implant. (See figure 9.)

Essentially, the microphone is an artificial eardrum. Instead of

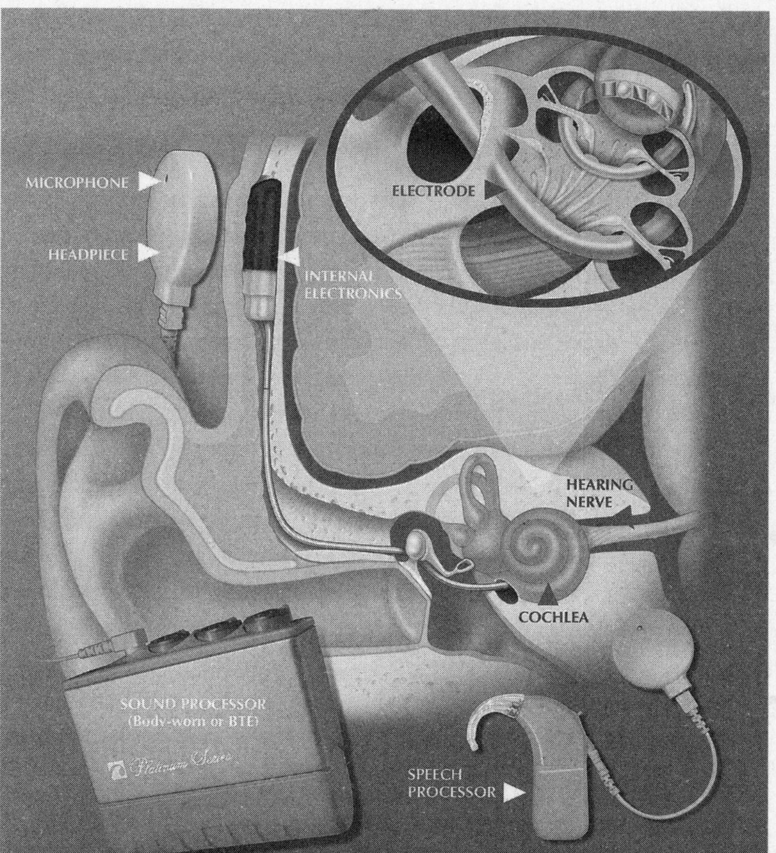

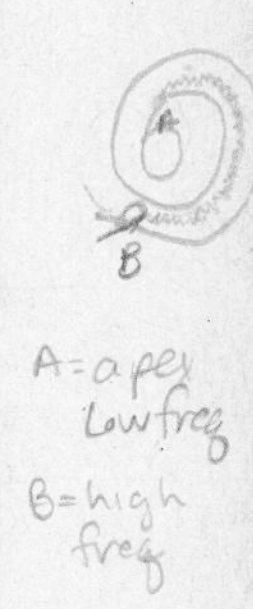

Figure 9. The internal and external components of a cochlear implant. The headpiece sticks to the head because both it and the implant have magnets in them, attracting each other through the skin. Two versions of the processor are shown: the waist-worn one with three controls, which is connected to the headpiece by a wire running under the shirt, and the one shaped like a hearing aid. Functionally, they are identical. The differences between them are of battery life and flexibility (the hearing-aid-shaped device has a smaller battery and only one control). In the close-up of the electrode array curled up in the cochlea, you can see the electrodes facing inward (the squares) and the silicone dividers separating them (the round dots). The electrode array fits into the lower of the cochlea's three chambers. The hair cells are in the smallest one. The electrode array literally bypasses the dead hair cells in order to stimulate the auditory nerves in the center of the cochlea.

skin, it is metal backed by a plastic plate. As the metal vibrates it induces a charge in the plastic, converting sound continuously into electricity. Cheryl's *O* will sweep on past the microphone as the milliseconds go by, reaching the walls beyond me, bouncing off them, reverberating, and finally fading into nothingness, but that will not matter: an electric charge is now propagating down the wire, faithfully preserving all of the information that was in the sound.

The electrical charge flows down the wire underneath my shirt to the computer at my belt. There it encounters an analog-to-digital converter, which dips a figurative finger into the river of electrons 17,000 times per second. Each time, it measures the volume and pitch and spews out numbers representing them. In goes a continuously flowing electric charge; out comes a digitized stream of numbers. And numbers can be manipulated. Indeed, that's all computers do, when you get right down to it: they shuffle numbers from one place to another. What we now have is a digital representation of the auditory world that can be sliced, diced, and puréed in any way a programmer might want.

Still inside the processor, the next step is to feed the numbers through the automatic gain control (AGC) subroutine, which squeezes the enormous range of sound that occurs in the natural world into a format that can be managed by the rest of the system. The difference in energy between the softest and the loudest sounds in human experience is surprisingly large. How much louder is a vacuum cleaner (80 dB) than a human voice (60 dB)? From looking at those numbers, you might think it was only 25 percent louder. Actually, it is *one hundred times* louder, in terms of how much physical energy there is in the sound wave emanating from it. The decibel system is logarithmic. An increase of 10 decibels is a tenfold increase in loudness; an increase of 20 dB is a hundredfold increase; of 30 dB, a thousandfold. Eighty dB is a hundred times louder than 60 dB, then. This is surprising to most people, because a vacuum cleaner doesn't *sound* one hundred times louder than a voice. It sounds maybe ten or twenty times louder. Conversely,

Cheryl's voice doesn't *sound* one hundred times fainter when she's ten feet away, even though it actually is. This is because the human ear has evolved to present a very cleverly manipulated auditory world to the brain. As explained in Chapter 5, when a small number of inner hair cells are triggered by a soft sound, the outer hair cells move in such a way that they cause *more* inner hair cells to fire. In effect, a soft sound triggers a cascading reaction that greatly increases how loud it seems to the listener. On the other end of the scale, extremely loud sounds trigger the *stapedius* muscle, which tightens so that the eardrum will move less; it's equivalent to your putting a finger on a loudspeaker to damp its vibration. The upshot is that you can hear both rustling leaves (10 dB) and a rock concert (110 dB), despite the fact that the former has *one ten-billionth* as much sound energy as the latter.* This is an extraordinary range compared to what most of the rest of your body can do; your muscles can't lift an ounce and also a thousand tons, and you can't walk both five miles an hour and a million. But you can hear sounds that are ten billion times softer than other sounds in your life. This flexibility accounts for why Cheryl's voice is still audible when its volume has dropped by a factor of a hundred, and why people can tolerate rock concerts that are hundreds of thousands of times louder than conversational speech.†

The engineers have to match this flexibility with software — at least partly. A 10 dB sound translates into an electrical stimulus of about a tenth of a milliamp. Any less electricity than that, and

* That is, 110 dB − 10 dB = a 100 dB difference, which is to say, a 10^{10} difference, which is to say, a difference of 10,000,000,000 (ten billion).

† The fact that a human ear can "tolerate" a rock concert doesn't mean that it should be asked to do so regularly. Over time, sound at high volume will damage the hair cells in the cochlea, starting with the ones that detect the high frequencies. It used to be thought that the damage simply came from sound waves battering the hair cells, but it is now known that the hair cells in fact *commit suicide.* Loud noises trigger a sequence of biochemical changes which lead inexorably to cell death. Research is now underway in developing drugs that interrupt that sequence to preserve hearing. There may come a day in the not-too-far future when musicians, factory workers, and military personnel may take a pill before noise exposure — sort of a sunscreen for the ears.

the nerves in the cochlea won't fire. Now let's say I walk into a rock concert where the noise level is 110 decibels, which as we've just seen is ten billion times louder than rustling leaves. If the system cranked up the electrical voltage proportionately, the wattage would be in the millions. That would melt the electrode array, fry my cochlea, explode my head, and markedly diminish the festivities (or maybe not, depending on the venue; according to Joe Quirk, such events would pass unnoticed at a Crash Worship gig). In reality, there isn't enough power in the rechargeable batteries powering the implant to actually do such a thing, but still, engineers take the idea of automatic gain control very seriously indeed. So the code fiddles with the numbers to ensure that the amount of electrical stimulation grows much more slowly than the energy level of the sound.

Once the AGC has had its way with the signal, it's shot along to the *bandpass filters,* which take sound apart for presentation to the auditory nerves. Each filter is programmed to pick out a different part of the frequency spectrum. Bandpass filter 1 isolates the lowest-frequency components, filter 2 the next-lowest, and so on depending on how many channels the system and its software can support. In my case, the system has 16 channels, thus there are 16 bandpass filters. (The filters consist purely of software manipulations of the numeric stream; they have no physical correlate anywhere in the chips.) Since the long *O* sound is mostly a low-frequency one, most of it is expressed by numbers streaming out of the low filters. A high-frequency sound, such as the rattling of keys, would be expressed mostly by the higher-frequency filters. Effectively, the computer is holding up 16 filters to the sound and getting 16 different versions of auditory reality.

The next step is to process the output of each bandpass filter through my *map.* Each user has different comfort levels at different electrodes. For example, users who have not heard high-frequency sounds in years may find high frequencies too sharp and piercing to bear, and therefore the audiologist will reduce the current levels in the high-frequency electrodes. Other users may have little nerve survival in particular places, so the audiologist may turn off the electrodes atop them so that their frequency information will be delivered to other places. Still others may find low-frequency sounds such as air-conditioning distracting, so the audiologist will turn them down or off altogether.

At this point, the system is ready to send the processed signal to the internal computer — "internal" meaning "inside my body." This is done by piping the binary data back up the cord to the headpiece, where our story began with the microphone. The obvious way to send information through unbroken skin is by radio waves, so the headpiece is a miniature radio transmitter, broadcasting the data to the implant using AM waves. It provides power as well. Electricity and radio are manifestations of the same underlying force and can readily be converted into each other. When electrons flow through a wire, some of the energy is dissipated as radio waves; conversely, when a radio signal encounters a wire, it generates a flow of electrons. The implant casing therefore contains a coil that not only picks up the radio signal but also generates enough electricity from it to power the chips and the electrode array.

The implant also beams radio signals back to the headpiece several times a second using a tiny FM transmitter, mostly to send "I am here and working fine" status reports to the processor. So the headpiece is a microphone and a magnet and an AM transmitter and an FM receiver.

While we're on the topic, there is one other way to get the information through the skin besides radio waves. You can punch a permanent hole in the skin, screw a titanium plug into the skull, and run a wire through it directly to the electrode array. There is no implant, no implant casing, no internal electronics. In the clipped language of biomedical engineers, this is called a *percutaneous* interface, "per" meaning "through" and "cutaneous" meaning "skin." Percutaneous interfaces have several advantages. There's no drain on energy from having to convert to radio and back, and there's no limits on bandwidth imposed by the physics of radio waves. Most of all, they're highly upgradable because all the computational

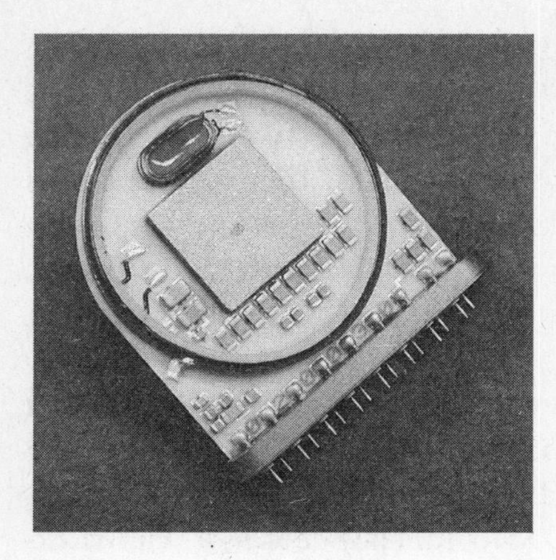

Figure 10. The reverse side of the implant (the front side is shown in figure 3). The large coil is the AM antenna; the small one is the FM transmitter. The metal square in the center is the magnet.

power is outside the body. Patients with percutaneous implants are much valued by researchers, because the electrode array can be controlled directly from the outside with no limitations whatsoever; any conceivable software can be tried on them. The Ineraid, the prototype implant used by Michael Pierschalla, was a percutaneous device.

However, the problems of percutaneous implants outweigh the advantages. Making a permanent hole in the skin invites bleeding and infection, and an impact in the right place can break the titanium plug right off (ow ow *owww*). There's also the safety problem inherent in having a wire running directly from the outside world into the body. An electrical shock could get conducted an inch and a half inside the user's head (also *ow*). And besides, a percutaneous interface is just plain creepy-looking. Not for nothing are most Borg implants percutaneous. Twenty-first-century biomedical engineers on Earth are more cautious: all commercial implants have *transcutaneous* interfaces, where radio waves convey the data through unbroken skin.

The electrode array is a series of tiny platinum plates embedded in a strip of silicone about an inch long and less than a millimeter wide. It's made by hand, and you can actually see that in a close-up look, because the plates are not quite exactly evenly spaced. A technician makes it while looking at it under a microscope, carefully laying out sixteen tiny wires, welding one to each plate, encasing the whole thing in silicone, and then painstakingly attaching each wire to one of the outputs of the implant. It's not easy work; it takes three months to train a technician to do the job, and finishing two a day is considered a good speed. The process could be automated, the engineers tell me, but it's not economical to spend millions of dollars to develop the machines to do so. Real efficiency in manufacturing electrode arrays may come with entirely new designs that use the same thin-film technology employed to fabricate computer chips. But, for now: handicraft.

Since the phoneme *O* is a low-frequency sound, it will be expressed mainly by firing the electrodes toward the end of the electrode array, where it rests closer to the apex of my cochlea. It has now been delivered to my auditory nerves, and the signal is creeping up my neural pathways to the brain. Each successive phoneme follows the *O* through the maze: the microphone, the analog-to-digital converter, the AGC, the bandpass filters, the map, the leap through the skin on radio waves, the reconversion into electricity, the reconstruction of the signal inside the implant, the firing of the electrode array. The whole process takes approximately four milliseconds. That is to say, I hear everything delayed by about four thousandths of a second. In human terms, this is no delay at all; I perceive myself hearing the word exactly as Cheryl speaks it.

During those four thousandths of a second, the falling acorn has moved a few millimeters closer to the ground; the waving hand is just a millimeter or two more extended now; the security gate's angle has increased just slightly to thirty-one degrees. The processor has gone through 131 more clock cycles, processing all those successive phonemes.

Okay, let's start time again.

"— *o*rning," Cheryl says to me.

I turn my head toward her as I walk past. It's a beautiful day. Between every footstep I take, my processor samples the world 8,500 times, executes 16 million instructions of code, and sends 556,818 ones and zeros into my head. My body is full of tiny etched silicon crystals computing away like mad. I know what animates my ear, I know the millions of clock cycles it executes every second to connect me to the world and the people I respect and love. The acorn hits the ground with a tiny *thump,* and an alert squirrel swivels his head and begins formulating plans to add it to his hoard for winter. The guard lowers his hand, and the security gate swings high to let one more person in for work. I know that the world is full of many fine marvelous things proceeding on all manner of time scales, beyond my ken; by such ceaseless activity does a universe constantly make and remake itself. I may carve out a life writing about as many of those things as time will allot me.

"Good *morning,*" I say back to Cheryl. And I smile.

NOTES

1. Broken

7 "The word is shorthand for *cyb*ernetic *org*anism, a term coined by Manfred Clynes and Nathan Kline": The definition of the word in their article "Cyborgs and Space" was rather more technical than WordNet's. "What are some of the devices necessary for creating self-regulating man-machine systems? This self-regulation must function without the benefit of consciousness in order to cooperate with the body's own autonomous homeostatic controls. For the exogenously extended organizational complex functioning as an integrated homeostatic system unconsciously, we propose the term 'Cyborg.' The Cyborg deliberately incorporates exogenous components extending the self-regulatory control function of the organism in order to adapt it to new environments" (pp. 30–31).

9 "To see is to observe, but to hear is to be enveloped": Hull, *Touching the Rock*, p. 83.

"They feel that it is *they* who have become unreal, not the world": In her memoir of getting a cochlear implant, Beverly Biderman writes, "Our environment has become dead, and we may also feel to some extent that we too have become dead. With my implant turned off, I feel like I am soundlessly walking down stairs and passing through rooms like a ghost." Biderman, *Wired for Sound*, p. 65.

10 "My misfortune is doubly painful to me": Beethoven, *The Heiligenstadt Testament*, online.

18 "Thou shalt not make a machine in the likeness of a man's mind": Herbert, *Dune*, p. 23.

"My very body would have technical specifications": These figures were provided to me by Mike Faltys and Logan Palmer of Advanced Bionics.

21 "You *are* a clumsy kid" and "Steve looked at him": Caidin, *Cyborg*, pp. 149 and 150.

2. Surgery

23 "Mothers in one Central African nation": Lane, *The Mask of Benevolence,* p. 11.

32 "a cohort of twenty thousand deaf children": CDC flyer, "Rubella (German Measles)," p. 1.

33 "And now I am becoming something else": I learned the details in this section by observing a cochlear implant surgery seven months after my own operation, thanks to the permission of Dr. Joseph Roberson, Becky Highlander, and Stanford Hospital. I have also drawn some of the details from Balkany, Cohen, and Gantz's article, "Surgical Technique for the Clarion Cochlear Implant."

35 "a plumber's snake passing through a curved drainpipe": Loeb, "The Functional Replacement of the Ear," p. 107.

"The problem preoccupied researchers for years": Clark, *Sounds from Silence,* p. 93.

37 "Human and human-made were brought together": Caidin, *Cyborg,* p. 119.

3. Between Two Worlds

40 "In one of the more egregious misuses of the word": Grossman, "Meet the Chipsons," pp. 56–57.

41 "If you have been technologically modified in any significant way": Gray, *Cyborg Citizen,* p. 2.

42 "he describes what his system can do": Mann, *Cyborg: Digital Destiny,* p. 203.

"Gregory Stock offers a more precise term": Stock, *Redesigning Humans,* pp. 24–25.

"Other theorists, such as Donna Haraway": See Haraway, "A Cyborg Manifesto."

44 "Its data transfer rate dropped from 134,000 bits per second": Jet Propulsion Laboratory, "This Week on Galileo," online.

45 "researchers have solemnly tabulated what various people hear": Griffiths, "Musical Hallucinosis," pp. 2065–2076.

46–47 "What thou lovest well is thy true heritage": Pound, *Canto LXXXI.*

5. Forget About Reality

67 "When I revisit that field in my mind's eye, I can see that it consists of fibers arranged in orderly rows": I am particularly indebted to two textbooks on hearing science, Pickles (1988) and Yost (2000), for much of the following information about the physiology of hearing. The animations offered at the University of Wisconsin–Madison's Web site, "Hearing and Balance" (http://www.neurophys.wisc.edu/h&b/auditory/fs-auditory

.html), greatly aided my understanding of auditory neural coding. The explanation of the decibel scale at "The Physics Classroom" (http://www.physicsclassroom.com/Class/sound/U11L2b.html) helped me understand the mathematics. Phillip Loizou's two tutorials on cochlear implants (1998, 1999) and Gerald Loeb's two articles on the implant's engineering and software (1985, 1996) were extremely helpful. Alex Alviar's astounding Web site, "Cochlear Implant Central," gave me a wealth of information on implant engineering and software. Conversations with Michael Dorman, Blake Wilson, Gerald Loeb, Charles Berlin, Phillip Loizou, Mike Faltys, Ed Overstreet, Kate Gfeller, Jay Rubinstein, Tony Spahr, Monita Chatterjee, Dewey Lawson, Reinhold Schatzer, Don Eddington, Robert Shannon, Susan Chorost, and many others helped me understand various terms and concepts.

68 "The outer hair cells receive signals *from* the brain": May, Budelis, and Niparko, "Behavioral Studies of the Olivocochlear Efferent System," p. 660.

72 "studies had shown that users broke more or less evenly given a choice between them": See Battmer, Zilberman, Haake, and Lenarz, "Simultaneous Analog Stimulation (SAS) — Continuous Interleaved Sampler (CIS) Pilot Comparison Study in Europe," and Osberger and Fisher, "SAS-CIS Preference Study in Postlingually Deafened Adults Implanted with the CLARION® Cochlear Implant."

6. The Computer Reprograms Me

82 "about 140,000 transistors": The numbers for my Clarion CII implant were provided by Logan Palmer, the chips' lead designer at Advanced Bionics. The number for the Intel 286 is from http://www.intel.com/pressroom/kits/quickreffam.htm#i486.

87–88 From "The brain is structured in such a way that it closely mirrors the body" to "Blind people who read Braille have been shown to have more brain surface devoted to the right index finger than do people with normal vision": Buonomano and Merzenich, "Cortical Plasticity," p. 168.

95 "Perversity, he suggested, comes from a pleasure-power complex": Foucault, *The History of Sexuality*, p. 48.

96 "He wanted to be rid of his unbearable humanity": Bettelheim, "Joey: A 'Mechanical Boy,'" p. 117.

97 "This recent film with this Terminator": In *The Cyborg Handbook*, ed. Gray, p. 47.

7. Upgrading

103 "Patients seem to do as well or better with replacement devices as they did before": See Fayad, Baino, Lee, and Parisier, "Cochlear Implant Reinser-

tion: Analysis and Outcome." They reviewed the charts of forty-five patients who had been reimplanted with new devices between 1982 and 2002 and found that speech recognition scores "remained stable or improved after reimplantation."

103 "In 1976 Graeme Clark, lead inventor of the Nucleus 22, had struggled to find $15,000 for a refrigerator-sized computer": Clark, *Sounds from Silence*, p. 57.

104–105 From "But in the late 1980s a group of engineers at Duke and Research Triangle Institution" to "Not perfectly, but much better than before": Wilson, "Strategies for Representing Speech," pp. 154–155.

107 "In 1978, Dr. Clark's first patient, Rod Saunders": Clark, *Sounds from Silence*, p. 113.

"The second patient's device failed ten months later": Clark, *Sounds from Silence*, p. 130.

108 Figure 8: "Speech Comprehension Improvement Over Time": Adapted from a chart given to me by Robert Shannon, House Ear Institute, Los Angeles, California.

110 "Researchers at Bell Labs showed, decades ago, that speech electronically filtered into a mere four channels was still intelligible to most listeners": Loizou, Dorman, and Tu, "On the Number of Channels Needed to Understand Speech," p. 2097. You can get an idea yourself of what the world sounds like when filtered into 1, 2, 4, 8, and 16 channels by going to http://www-rohan.sdsu.edu/~aboothro/files/ and clicking on "Implant Simulations.ppt." This is only an approximation of what the world sounds like through a cochlear implant, because a cochlear implant changes far more aspects of the auditory system than just its number of channels. However, listening to the difference between 8 and 16 channels can give you some idea of the difference between SAS/CIS and Hi-Res.

115 "The cyborg is resolutely committed to partiality, irony, intimacy, and perversity": Haraway, "A Cyborg Manifesto," p. 151.

8. The Logic I Loved and Hated

117 "Why do you test for humans?": Herbert, *Dune*, p. 23.

119 "This is scoping, San Francisco–style": Kapp, "Generation Single," p. 55.

"When a person has, say, just five choices": Schwartz, "The Tyranny of Choice," p. 73.

121 "reached the same linguistic performance range as normally hearing children after six months": McConkey Robbins et al., "Effect of Age at Cochlear Implantation on Auditory Skill Development in Infants and Toddlers."

"In a study of 181 children who received cochlear implants in the mid-1990s": Geers, "Speech, Language, and Reading Skills," p. 634.

123 "Ninety-six percent of the deaf children born in the United States are born to parents with normal hearing": Mitchell and Karchmer, "Chasing the Mythical Ten Percent," p. 22.

"a safe and effective technology": In a study of 733 cochlear implant surgeries between 1993 and 2002, the postoperative infection rate was found to be 4.1 percent. The authors conclude, "Cochlear implants remain a safe procedure with a low complication rate." Cunningham, Slattery, and Luxford, "Postoperative Infection in Cochlear Implant Patients."

127 "In a study of sixty-five children with cochlear implants, an astonishing 60 percent of them were said by their parents to enjoy music and seek it out": Gfeller et al., "Musical Involvement and Enjoyment of Children Who Use Cochlear Implants," p. 223.

"When so much of the world is indecipherable": Cohen, *Train Go Sorry*, p. 7.

128 "Have you ever come into our World?": This entry was at http://members.aol.com/_ht_a/SCarter11/gd1.htm when I accessed it on September 7, 2002. It no longer seems to be available.

"TV and air-conditioning went on the market just four years apart": Putnam, *Bowling Alone*, p. 217.

"Between 1974 and 1994 the number of Americans serving as an officer of some club or organization dropped by 42 percent": Putnam, *Bowling Alone*, p. 45.

129 "Even less formal activities — ones we associate with simple friendship and community — have declined precipitously": Putnam, *Bowling Alone*, p. 99. The source of such fine-grained information is organizations such as the Roper poll, which once a month asked thousands of Americans to say which of a given list of activities they had engaged in during the past year (Putnam, p. 40).

130 "A position statement released by the National Association for the Deaf . . . in 1991": I have not been able to find the statement either online or in print, although the phrase "cultural genocide" is widely remembered.

131 "Sign language was suppressed": Lane, *The Mask of Benevolence*, pp. 113 and 117.

132 "The NAD . . . respects their choice to use cochlear implants": National Association for the Deaf, "Position Statement," online.

"It seems to us that the walls between those who support pediatric implantation and those who oppose the procedure are, if not crumbling . . .": Christiansen and Leigh, *Cochlear Implants in Children*, p. 321.

132–133 "In 2000, however, 59 percent of Gallaudet's faculty, staff, and students questioned in a poll agreed that the school should do more to encourage students with cochlear implants to attend": Christiansen and Leigh, *Cochlear Implants in Children*, p. 283.

133 "Heather Artinian, got a cochlear implant in September 2002": *Good Morning America,* telecast April 29, 2003.

"In a documentary of a child with a cochlear implant": Advanced Bionics, *Cecilia's Story,* 2002.

"A group of seventeen- and eighteen-year-old deaf students studied by Gallaudet researchers in 1997 had a median reading ability at a fourth-grade level": Gallaudet Research Institute, "Literacy & Deaf Students," online.

135 "Figures gathered by Gallaudet bear out a growing suspicion that race is an important factor in who gets an implant": Christiansen and Leigh, *Cochlear Implants in Children,* p. 328.

"Demographics collected by Gallaudet show that of the 42,361 students in the United States with hearing losses on which they collected data": Gallaudet Research Institute, *Regional and National Summary Report of Data from the 2001–2002 Annual Survey of Deaf and Hard of Hearing Children & Youth,* p. 1.

"One study compared 816 profoundly deaf children with cochlear implants to 816 profoundly deaf children without implants": Holden-Pitt, "Who and Where Are Our Children with Cochlear Implants?," slides 5 and 9.

"Why do so many fewer minority children get cochlear implants than white children? I put this question to José Blackorby": Interview with Dr. José Blackorby, SRI International, Menlo Park, California. Conducted May 28, 2004.

136 "Already poor, with over 50 percent unemployment": U.S. Census Bureau, "Survey of Income and Program Participation," p. 8.

9. A Kinship with the Machines

147 "The cyborg would not recognize the Garden of Eden": Haraway, "A Cyborg Manifesto," p. 151.

148 "The cyborg is a creature in a post-gender world": Haraway, "A Cyborg Manifesto," p. 150.

153 "Single vision produces worse illusions": Haraway, "A Cyborg Manifesto," p. 154.

155 "A cyborg body is not innocent": Haraway, "A Cyborg Manifesto," p. 180.

"From another perspective, a cyborg world": Haraway, "A Cyborg Manifesto," p. 154.

10. A Kinship with the Humans

160 "He'd sent me one of his articles several months before": Loeb et al., "Design and Fabrication of an Experimental Cochlear Prosthesis."

167 "out of tens of thousands of implant surgeries worldwide, ninety-one cases and seventeen deaths had been reported, with U.S. numbers being

twenty-nine and three, respectively": The worldwide figures come from Hagan, "Falling on Deaf Ears," *New Scientist,* p. 38. The U.S. figures come from Cohen, Roland, and Marrinan, "Meningitis in Cochlear Implant Recipients: The North American Experience," p. 276.

168 "Lee and Stone had coauthored a paper": Moore et al., "Dual Action Automatic Gain Control System in a Cochlear Implant," poster session, CIAP 1999.

11. The Technologies of Human Potential

172 "the House Ear Institute in L.A. has developed a computerized training system": Qian-Jie Fu et al., "CAST: An Auditory Rehabilitation Tool for Cochlear Implant Patients," poster session, CIAP 2003.

173 "the auditory cortex of musicians is 130 percent larger than that of nonmusicians, and children exposed to music early in life": Weinberger, "Music and the Brain," *Scientific American,* p. 94.

175 "Human communication is on the verge of a complete overhaul": Warwick, *I, Cyborg,* p. 3.

176 "With the interlinking of human and machine brains . . . it should be possible, within the next fifteen years, to upgrade memory . . .": Warwick, *I, Cyborg,* p. 295.

"A company called Cyberkinetics is designing 'brain implant' chips": Pollack, "With Tiny Brain Implants," section F, page 5.

"Similar work is being done by Duke University's Miguel Nicolelis, who has trained monkeys to move artificial arms by mental signals — that is, by thinking": Reuters, "Thought-control Experiments," online.

177 "I told everyone that this would ultimately mean . . . we should be able to drive a car around by picking up the signals directly from the brain": Warwick, *I, Cyborg,* p. 235.

179 "five frequently mentioned obstacles that many experts had considered insuperable": Clark, *Sounds from Silence,* p. 54.

180 "In medieval times, a skilled troubadour needed to hear a long poem recited only three times": Burke, *The Day the Universe Changed,* p. 98.

"Mnemonic techniques such as the 'memory palace,' where people memorized information by situating it in a visualized physical space": See Yates, *The Art of Memory.*

181 "Putnam estimates that television *alone* accounts for about 25 percent of the decline": Putnam, *Bowling Alone,* p. 283. Putnam suggests that about 50 percent of the decline is due to generational change, the inexorable replacement of a generation of "joiners" and "schmoozers" with their less civic-minded children and grandchildren. But this is a demographic phenomenon rather than a cause in and of itself.

"Dependence on television for entertainment is not merely *a* significant predictor of civic disengagement": Putnam, *Bowling Alone,* p. 231.

182 "It may seem contrary to intuition": Mann, *Cyborg: Digital Destiny,* p. 211.

"The solution will be to find ways": Mann, *Cyborg: Digital Destiny,* p. 211.

12. Mike 2.0

188 "We have put between ourselves and the natural world": Birkerts, *Readings,* p. 7.

191 "For I am now, after forty years of what we will term silence": Wright, *Deafness,* p. 12.

Appendix

199 "Thus I too must praise out of a quiet ear": Wright, *Deafness,* p. 3.

"The cochlea operates as a short-term Fourier analyzer": Palmer, "Neural Signal Processing," p. 75.

BIBLIOGRAPHY

Advanced Bionics. *Cecilia's Story.* Sylmar, California: Advanced Bionics, 2002.

Alexandre, Daniel, and Alain Ghysen. "Somatotopy of the Lateral Line Projection in Larval Zebrafish." *Proceedings of the National Academy of Sciences of the USA* 96:13 (June 22, 1999): 7558–7562. Available at http://www.pubmedcentral.nih.gov/articlerender.fcgi?artid=22125#B4.

Alviar, Alex. "Cochlear Implant Central." Available at http://www.geocities.com/cicentral.

Aronson, Josh (director). *Sound and Fury.* New York: New Video Group, 2000.

Balkany, Thomas J., Noel L. Cohen, and Bruce J. Gantz. "Surgical Technique for the Clarion Cochlear Implant." *Annals of Otology, Rhinology & Laryngology* 108:4 (April 1999): 27–30.

Battmer, Rolf D., Yitzak Zilberman, Philip Haake, and Thomas Lenarz. "Simultaneous Analog Stimulation (SAS) — Continuous Interleaved Sampler (CIS) Pilot Comparison Study in Europe." *Annals of Otology, Rhinology & Laryngology* 108:4 (April 1999): 69–73.

Beethoven, Ludwig van. "The Heiligenstadt Testament, for My Brothers Carl and Johann Beethoven." Available at http://www.maurice-abravanel.com/beethoven_testament.html. Accessed March 8, 2004.

Bettelheim, Bruno. "Joey: A 'Mechanical Boy.'" *Scientific American,* March 1959: 116–127. Reprinted in *The Uncanny: Experiments in Cyborg Culture,* Bruce Grenville, ed. Vancouver: Arsenal Pulp Press, 2002.

Biderman, Beverly. *Wired for Sound: A Journey into Hearing.* Toronto: Trifolium Books, 1998.

Birkerts, Sven. *Readings.* Saint Paul, Minn.: Graywolf Press, 1999.

Buonomano, Dean V., and Michael M. Merzenich. "Cortical Plasticity: From Synapses to Maps." *Annual Review of Neuroscience* 21 (1998): 149–186.

Burke, James. *The Day the Universe Changed: How Galileo's Telescope Changed the Truth and Other Events in History That Dramatically Altered Our Understanding of the World.* New York: Back Bay Books, 1995.

Burke, Kenneth. *The Philosophy of Literary Form*. Berkeley: University of California Press, 1974.

Caidin, Martin. *Cyborg*. New York: Warner Paperback Library, 1972.

Castaneda, Carlos. *The Teachings of Don Juan: A Yaqui Way of Knowledge*. New York: Simon and Schuster, 1968.

Centers for Disease Control and Prevention. "Rubella (German Measles)." Available at http://www.cdc.gov/nip/publications/Parents-Guide/pg-rubella.pdf.

Chorost, Michael. "Hearing Ear, Hearing I." *Journal of the Academy of Rehabilitative Audiology* 31 (Spring 1998): 123–130.

Christiansen, John B., and Irene W. Leigh. *Cochlear Implants in Children: Ethics and Choices*. Washington, D.C.: Gallaudet University Press, 2002.

Clark, Andy. *Natural-Born Cyborgs: Minds, Technologies, and the Future of Human Intelligence*. Oxford: Oxford University Press, 2003.

Clark, Graeme. *Sounds from Silence: Graeme Clark and the Bionic Ear Story*. Sydney, Australia: Allen & Unwin, 2000.

Clynes, Manfred, and Nathan Kline. "Cyborgs and Space." Originally published in *Astronautics*, September 1960. In *The Cyborg Handbook*, Chris Hables Gray, ed. New York: Routledge, 1995.

Cohen, Leah Hager. *Train Go Sorry: Inside a Deaf World*. New York: Vintage Books, 1995.

Cohen, Noel L., Thomas Roland, Jr., and Michelle Marrinan. "Meningitis in Cochlear Implant Recipients: The North American Experience." *Otology and Neurotology* 25 (May 2004): 275–281.

Cunningham, Calhoun D., William H. Slattery, and William M. Luxford. "Postoperative Infection in Cochlear Implant Patients." *Archives of Otolaryngology — Head and Neck Surgery* 131 (July 2004): 109–114.

Dennett, Daniel C. *Consciousness Explained*. Boston: Little, Brown and Company, 1991.

Dibbell, Julian. *My Tiny Life: Crime and Passion in a Virtual World*. New York: Henry Holt, 1999. The chapter from which I quote is available online at http://www.juliandibbell.com/texts/bungle.html.

Fayad, J. N., T. E. Baino, D. Lee, and S. C. Parisier. "Cochlear Implant Reinsertion: Analysis and Outcome." Proceedings of the *Cochlear Implants in Children 2003* Conference, Washington D.C., April 24, 2003.

Foucault, Michel. *The History of Sexuality, Volume 1*. New York: Vintage Books, 1980.

Fu, Qian-Jie, John Galvin III, Xiaosong Wang, and Geri Nogaki. "CAST: An Auditory Rehabilitation Tool for Cochlear Implant Patients." Poster session, Conference for Implantable Auditory Prostheses, Asilomar, California, August 17–22, 2003.

Gallaudet Research Institute. "Literacy & Deaf Students." Washington, D.C.: Gallaudet University, October 2003. Available at http://gri.gallaudet.edu/Literacy.

Gallaudet Research Institute. *Regional and National Summary Report of Data from the 2001–2002 Annual Survey of Deaf and Hard of Hearing Children & Youth.* Washington, D.C.: Gallaudet University, January 2003. Available at http://gri.gallaudet.edu/Demographics/2002_National_Summary.pdf.

Geers, Ann E. "Speech, Language, and Reading Skills After Early Cochlear Implantation." *Archives of Otolaryngology — Head and Neck Surgery* 130 (May 2004): 634–638.

Gfeller, Kate, Shelley A. Witt, Linda J. Spencer, Julie Stordahl, and Bruce Tomblin. "Musical Involvement and Enjoyment of Children Who Use Cochlear Implants." *The Volta Review* 100:4 (2000): 213–233.

Good Morning America. Story on the Artinian family, telecast date April 29, 2003. Transcript available from http://www.transcripts.tv/good-morning-america.cfm (locate it by searching the archive for "Artinian").

Gray, Chris Hables. *Cyborg Citizen: Politics in the Posthuman Age.* New York and London: Routledge, 2002.

Griffiths, T. D. "Musical Hallucinosis in Acquired Deafness." *Brain* 123 (2000): 2065–2076.

Grossman, Lev. "Meet the Chipsons." *Time,* March 11, 2002, 56–57.

Hagan, Pat. "Falling on Deaf Ears." *New Scientist,* August 28, 2004, 36–39.

Haraway, Donna. "A Cyborg Manifesto: Science, Technology, and Socialist-Feminism in the Late Twentieth Century." In *Simians, Cyborgs and Women: The Reinvention of Nature.* London: Free Association Books, 1991. This essay is widely available on the Internet, for example, at http://www.stanford.edu/dept/HPS/Haraway/CyborgManifesto.html.

Herbert, Frank. *Dune.* London: New English Library, 1965.

Holden-Pitt, Lisa. "Who and Where Are Our Children with Cochlear Implants?" Paper presented at the American Speech-Language-Hearing Association (ASHA), Boston, Massachusetts, November 20–23, 1997. Available at http://gri.gallaudet.edu/Cochlear/ASHA.1997/index.html.

Hull, John M. *Touching the Rock: An Experience of Blindness.* New York: Pantheon, 1990.

Jet Propulsion Laboratory. "This Week on Galileo." October 8, 2000, 276–282. Available at http://galileo.jpl.nasa.gov/news/thiswk/today001002.html. Accessed January 1, 2004.

Kapp, Diana. "Generation Single." *San Francisco,* February 2004, 52–59.

Lane, Harlan. *The Mask of Benevolence.* 2nd ed. New York: Dawn Sign Press, 1999.

Loeb, G. E., C. L. Byers, S. J. Rebscher, D. E. Casey, M. M. Fong, R. A. Schindler, R. F. Gray, and M. M. Merzenich. "Design and Fabrication of an Experimental Cochlear Prosthesis." *Medical & Biological Engineering & Computing* 21 (May 1983): 241–254.

Loeb, Gerald. "The Functional Replacement of the Ear." *Scientific American* 252:2 (February 1985): 104–110.

Loeb, Gerald. "An Information Highway to the Auditory Nerve." *Seminars in Hearing* 17:4 (November 1996): 309–316.

Loizou, Phillip. "Mimicking the Human Ear." *IEEE Signal Processing Magazine* 15:5 (September 1998): 101–130.

Loizou, Phillip. "Introduction to Cochlear Implants." *IEEE Engineering in Medicine and Biology,* January/February 1999: 32–42.

Loizou, Phillip, Michael Dorman, and Zhemin Tu. "On the Number of Channels Needed to Understand Speech." *Journal of the Acoustical Society of America* 106:4 (October 1999): 2097–2103.

Mann, Steve, with Hal Niedzviecki. *Cyborg: Digital Destiny and Human Possibility in the Age of the Wearable Computer.* Toronto: Doubleday Canada, 2002.

May, Bradford J., Jennifer Budelis, and John K. Niparko. "Behavioral Studies of the Olivocochlear Efferent System: Learning to Listen in Noise." *Archives of Otolaryngology — Head and Neck Surgery* 130 (May 2004): 660–664.

McConkey Robbins, Amy, Dawn Burton Koch, Mary Joe Osberger, Susan Zimmerman-Phillips, and Liat Kishon-Rabin. "Effect of Age at Cochlear Implantation on Auditory Skill Development in Infants and Toddlers." *Archives of Otolaryngology — Head and Neck Surgery* 130 (May 2004): 570–574.

Mitchell, Ross E., and Michael A. Karchmer. "Chasing the Mythical Ten Percent: Parental Hearing Status of Deaf and Hard of Hearing Students in the United States." *Sign Language Studies* 4:2 (Winter 2004): 138–163. Also available from Gallaudet Research Institute's Web site at http://gri.gallaudet.edu/Demographics/SLS_Paper.pdf.

Moore, Brian C. J., Stanley Chim, Michael Stone, and Jason Lee. "Dual Action Automatic Gain Control System in a Cochlear Implant." Conference on Implantable Auditory Prostheses 1999, Poster Session #4, Asilomar, California, August 29–September 3, 1999. Abstract available at http://www.iupui.edu/~iuoto/asilomar/1999/ciap99postersess4.html.

National Association for the Deaf. "NAD Position Statement on Cochlear Implants." October 2000. Available at the NAD Web site, http://www.nad.org/infocenter/newsroom/positions/CochlearImplants.html.

Osberger, Mary Joe, and Laurel Fisher. "SAS-CIS Preference Study in Postlingually Deafened Adults Implanted with the CLARION® Cochlear Implant." *Annals of Otology, Rhinology & Laryngology* 108:4 (April 1999): 74–79.

Palmer, Alan R. "Neural Signal Processing." In *Hearing,* C. J. Moore, ed. San Diego: Academic Press, 1995.

Pickles, James O. *An Introduction to the Physiology of Hearing.* 2nd ed. London: Academic Press, 1988.

Pollack, Andrew. "With Tiny Brain Implants, Just Thinking May Make It So." *New York Times,* April 13, 2004, section F, page 5.

Pound, Ezra. "Canto LXXXI." In the *Norton Anthology of Modern Poetry,* Richard Ellmann and Robert O'Clair, eds. New York: W. W. Norton & Co., 1973: 367–371.

Putnam, Robert D. *Bowling Alone: The Collapse and Revival of American Community.* New York: Simon & Schuster, 2000.

Reuters. "Thought-Control Experiments May Benefit Parkinson's Patients." March 24, 2004. Available at http://www.abc.net.au/news/newsitems/s1072740.htm.

Rich, Adrienne. *Poems: Selected and New, 1950–1974.* New York: W. W. Norton & Company, 1975.

Romoff, Arlene. *Hear Again: Back to Life with a Cochlear Implant.* New York: League for the Hard of Hearing, 1999.

Schwartz, Barry. "The Tyranny of Choice." *Scientific American* 290 (April 2004): 70–75.

Stock, Gregory. *Redesigning Humans: Choosing Our Genes, Changing Our Future.* Boston: Mariner Books, 2003.

U.S. Census Bureau, 1997. Survey of Income and Program Participation tables. Available at http://www.census.gov/hhes/www/disable/emperndistbl.pdf.

Waldrop, Judith, and Sharon M. Stern. "Disability Status: 2000." U.S. Census, 2000 (March 2003). Available at http://www.census.gov/prod/2003 pubs/c2kbr-17.pdf.

Warwick, Kevin. *I, Cyborg.* London: Century, 2002.

Weinberger, Norman M. "Music and the Brain." *Scientific American* 290 (November 2004): 89–95.

Weizenbaum, Joseph. *Computer Power and Human Reason: From Judgment to Calculation.* San Francisco: W. H. Freeman and Company, 1976.

Wilson, Blake S. "Strategies for Representing Speech with Cochlear Implants." In *Cochlear Implants: Principles and Practices,* John K. Niparko, ed. Philadelphia: Lippincott Williams & Wilkins, 2000.

Wright, David. *Deafness.* New York: Stein and Day, 1969.

Yates, Francis. *The Art of Memory.* Chicago: University of Chicago Press, 1966.

Yost, William A. *Fundamentals of Hearing: An Introduction.* 4th ed. San Diego: Academic Press, 2000.

ACKNOWLEDGMENTS

A great many scientists and engineers patiently answered my questions and read portions of the manuscript for accuracy. I thank Chuck Berlin, Gerald Loeb, Michael Merzenich, Michael Dorman, Curtis Ponton, Anthony Spahr, Phillip Loizou, Jay Rubinstein, Blake Wilson, Dewey Lawson, Reinhold Schatzer, Amy McConkey Robbins, Don Eddington, Robert Shannon, Sig Soli, Kate Gfeller, Susan Waltzman, Beverly Wright, Bernd Fritzsch, Jim Patrick, Eric Lynch, and Bob White. All responsibility for errors, of course, is mine alone.

The manufacturer of my implant, Advanced Bionics, gave me incredible assistance at every step of the way. I am very grateful for the help given me by Van Harrison, Doug Lynch, Mike Faltys, Tracey Kruger, Patricia Trautwein, Thomas Santogrossi, Albert Maltan, Mike Brownen, Dorcas Kessler, Leo Litvak, Logan Palmer, Ed Overstreet, Julie French, Todd Foster, and Carla Woods.

Thanks to Dr. Joseph Roberson of the California Ear Institute, whose skilled hands put my new ear in place; to Becky Highlander, who programmed and reprogrammed me with endless patience; and to Cache Pitt, Bruna Gasparini, and Dr. Ted Mason, for additional audiological, medical, and photographic support.

For pitch-perfect editing and moral support, I thank my fellow writers Tamim Ansary, Cheyenne Richards, Scott James, Maria Strom, Rob Tocalino, Cheryl Dahle, Martha Engber, Ken Grosserode, Annika Wood, and not least, Joe Quirk. Other people who read parts of the manuscript and gave me encouragement are Linda Shear, Camille Marder, Marcelo Hoffman, Louise Yarnall, Jennifer Cumming, Paula Rosenthal, Janice Y.

Song, Alex Alviar, and Janet Alviar. For helping me brainstorm the title, I thank Pam Burdman, who helped me generate at least two hundred titles in one evening. This was a very difficult book to title.

I thank Arlene Romoff and Beverly Biderman, authors of *Hear Again* and *Wired for Sound*, for writing of their own experiences with their cochlear implants. I reread both of their books several times before and after activation, and they helped greatly in guiding me through the experience.

I'm very grateful to my supervisors at SRI International, who gave me extraordinary behind-the-scenes support while I was laboring to get this book written. I could not have written this book without the time and breathing room they gave me. My deep thanks to Gary Bridges, Peter Ryan, José Blackorby, and Dennis Beatrice. Thanks also to Cheryl Villavicencio and Amy Wallace, who made phone calls for me for three months.

For information on Michael Pierschalla's life and untimely death, I thank Martha Woodworth, who sent me his letters and diaries.

I thank Elsevier, the parent corporation of Academic Press, for giving me permission to reproduce the electron micrographs of hair cells shown in Chapter 5, and James O. Pickles, the author of *An Introduction to the Physiology of Hearing*, for sending me high-quality electronic versions of them.

Thanks to the women I have dated, all of whom have reviewed the sections about them and bravely given me permission to use the material. Their names have been changed, but my gratitude for their companionship has not. To Claire Cotts, thanks for the inspired suggestion of "Steve Austin seeks Jane Austen" as my Salon Personals tagline.

I want to thank one person whom I have never known and never will. This book was profoundly influenced by David Wright's beautifully written memoir, *Deafness*. In many ways this book is a sequel to his, picking up many of his themes and recasting them in an age dominated by the computer. Had I been born in 1920, my life could have been very much like his. And had he been born in 1964, his life could have been very much like mine. I like to think that if he had published *Deafness* in 2005 rather than 1969, it would have been this book.

I am honored to thank Sol Stein for his help with my book proposal and his advice on many other publishing-related matters. He was the publisher of the American edition of David Wright's *Deafness.* I can only view it as pure karma that he is also my father's next-door neighbor.

It took me three years to write this book, but I had been thinking about many of its ideas since 1993 when I took a course taught by Cathy Davidson at Duke University and wrote a term paper entitled "Cyborg Ear, Cyborg I." She was the first person to suggest that I consider expanding it into a book. Twelve years later, her suggestion has borne fruit. Thanks to Linda Thibodeau, my audiologist at UT-Austin and editor of the *Journal of the Academy of Rehabilitative Audiology,* which published a short article of mine in 1998 that also contained some of the ideas developed in this book. I also want to thank Barbara Herrnstein Smith at Duke and Michele Jackson at the University of Colorado for helping me brainstorm some of the literary-theoretical ideas in this book. Last but not least, deep thanks to John Slatin, my dissertation chair at UT-Austin, who in teaching me how to write a dissertation also taught me how to write this book.

Deep thanks go to Michael Carlisle, my agent, and my editors at Houghton Mifflin, Laura van Dam and Amanda Cook. They took a huge chance on an unknown first-time author. For their constant faith and superb guidance, I am more grateful than I can say. I also thank Larry Chilnick and Ted Weinstein, book people extraordinaire, for their encouragement and good advice, and Erica Avery, Beth Fuller, and Pilar Queen for capable behind-the-scenes support.

To Jeff Weill, David Chioni Moore, Heather Johnson, Marie and Matthew Troidl, Kristin Bosetti, Shoshana Billik, Elizabeth Vander Schaaf, Margaret Pak, Paula Tanksley, and Wendy Besterman, my enduring thanks for your friendship.

Finally, thanks inexpressible to Susan Chorost and Sherwood Chorost, also known as Mom and Dad, for their help in more ways than I can possibly count while writing this book.

INDEX